Anxiety Relief

Mindfulness Strategy for Kids and Teens With Adhd

(A Comprehensive Guide to Navigate the Lifelong Journey and Overcoming Anxiety)

William Eldredge

Published By **Gautam Kumar**

William Eldredge

Anxiety Relief: Mindfulness Strategy for Kids and Teens With Adhd (A Comprehensive Guide to Navigate the Lifelong Journey and Overcoming Anxiety)

ISBN 978-1-7753927-5-0

Legal & Disclaimer

Table Of Contents

Chapter 1: What Is Anxiety?

Anxiety is a commonplace and often healthful emotion. It is the body's everyday response to chance or strain. When we're stressful, our systems release hormones which embody adrenaline and cortisol, which put together us to combat or run.

Anxiety can be produced through a large number of reasons, each actual and perceived. Common triggers encompass:

Stressful existence activities, which embody task loss, divorce, or infection

Financial issues

Work or faculty stress

Relationship issues

Social activities

Health problems

Medical methods

Past bad occurrences

Anxiety can emerge in some of methods, both bodily and emotional. Common symptoms consist of:

Restlessness

Feeling tight or uncomfortable

Rapid heartbeat

Sweating

Shallow breathing

Difficulty concentrating

Difficulty napping

Fatigue

Headaches

Stomachaches

Muscle anxiety

Panic attacks

In sure conditions, tension may be so acute that it interferes with each day lifestyles. When this takes place, it is essential to looking for professional treatment.

Why do teenagers revel in Anxiety?

Teens suffer tension for an entire lot of motives. Some of the most regular motives encompass:

Brain improvement: The teenage mind remains growing, and the portions of the mind that manipulate feelings and impulse manipulate are not yet certainly mature. This should make young adults extra sensitive to fear.

Hormonal adjustments: Puberty is a time of excellent hormonal adjustments, which can also cause worry.

Increased stress: Teens enjoy several pressures, every at college and at home. These pressures can embody instructional pressure, social stress, and family problems.

Perfectionism: Many kids are perfectionists, and they installation high desires for themselves. This can result in anxiety, particularly when they sense like they'll be now not conducting their wishes.

Social media: Social media may be a purpose of fear for young adults, as they enjoy pressure to evaluate themselves to others and to task an ideal photo on line.

Mental fitness records: Teens who've a circle of relatives records of intellectual contamination are more likely to boom anxiety themselves.

Here are some particular instances of events which could provoke tension in teenagers:

School: Tests, shows, peer stress, bullying

Social: Dating, gatherings, public talking

Family: Parental war, divorce, infection in the circle of relatives

Health: Medical techniques, continual ailment, frame photo troubles

World occasions: Violence, terrorism, political instability

It is vital to recognition on that anxiety is a everyday problem of existence, and everyone research it every now and then. However, if anxiety is powerful or chronic, it'd intrude with each day existence. If you're involved that your youngster may be struggling with with tension, please obtain out to a intellectual fitness professional for assist.

How may additionally moreover this e-book gain you?

This e-book assist you to in numerous methods, together with:

Teaching you approximately the neurobiology of anxiety: This can will assist you to recognize why you experience anxiety and the manner to retrain your thoughts to answer lots much less nervously.

Providing you with fun techniques: These methods can permit you to alleviate stress and tension in the gift.

Teaching you a way to control tough feelings healthily: This will allow you to cope with tension-related feelings which include fear, worry, and depression.

Teaching you a manner to hit upon and confront horrible beliefs: This will will let you adjust the way you recollect anxiety and establish more useful and realistic thoughts.

Teaching you a manner to deal with avoidant dispositions: This will will will let you face your worries and stay a more captivating existence.

In addition to the foregoing, this e-book additionally offers you self-assessment questions, an workout/skill index, and an index. This will permit you to tune your development, choose out regions in that you need greater help, and accumulate the records and property you want.

Chapter 2: You Can Retrain Your Brain

The amygdala is a tiny almond-usual location within the mind that plays a essential function in processing worry and tension. When we encounter a risk, the amygdala sends a sign to the rest of the body, prompting the combat-or-flight reaction. This is a natural and wholesome response, however it can become difficult whilst it is delivered on too without difficulty or too frequently.

The suitable news is that you could retrain your amygdala to respond an awful lot a lot much less nervously. This manner is called neuroplasticity, and it refers to the brain's potential to regulate and adapt in response to new studies.

One approach to rewire your amygdala is through publicity treatment. Exposure remedy includes step by step exposing oneself to the matters which you fear in a stable and controlled environment. Over time, this allows your amygdala to investigate that the ones objects are not truly dangerous, and the fight-or-flight reaction is a good deal much less probable to be brought on.

Another technique to reprogramming your amygdala is thru mindfulness. By concentrating hobby at the prevailing 2d without passing judgment, mindfulness is practiced. When you're aware, you can note your thoughts and emotions with out turning into stuck up in them. This can can help you end up more privy to your anxiety triggers and to create more useful coping strategies.

Here are a few unique sports activities sports that you may do to retrain your amygdala:

Exposure remedy

Make a listing of the matters that you worry, ranked from least to maximum feared.

Start via exposing yourself to the least frightened aspect on your listing. This want to require genuinely thinking about the object, or it could contain frequently exposing yourself to it in actual life.

Once you're comfortable with the least feared object, circulate immediately to the following object in your listing.

Continue this method till you have exposed yourself to all the devices to your listing.

Mindfulness

Find a peaceful vicinity wherein you'll no longer be .

Close your eyes on the same time as you're taking a seat in a snug feature.

Bring your interest on your breath. Notice the sensation of your breath stepping into and exiting your frame.

When your mind wanders, lightly bring it again to your breath.

Continue this exercise for 5-10 minutes every day.

It is essential to be slight with your self at the same time as retraining your amygdala. It takes time and exercise to trade your mind's response to worry and anxiety. However, with regular artwork, you may discover ways to manipulate your anxiety and live a happier and more healthy existence.

Here are a few hints for achievement:

Start carefully and progressively growth the problem of your exposures.

Make certain that your exposures are completed in a safe and managed environment.

Find a nice therapist or counselor who permit you to at the facet of your exposure treatment.

Be patient and constant alongside facet your mindfulness exercise.

If you are suffering to retrain your amygdala in your private, please attain out to a intellectual health expert for assist.

What is the amygdala?

The amygdala is a tiny, almond-shaped place within the thoughts that performs a essential function in processing fear and anxiety. It is positioned within the temporal lobe, proper now at the back of the hippocampus. The amygdala is part of the limbic machine, a network of thoughts regions which can be involved in emotion, motivation, and memory.

The amygdala gets sensory input from all of the senses, and it's miles specifically sensitive to visible and auditory cues which are associated with chance. When the amygdala acknowledges a capability hazard, it sends indicators to the rest of the mind, prompting the fight-or-flight response. This is a natural and healthy reaction that permits us to live on in tough situations.

However, the amygdala can from time to time be overactive, allowing us to experience dread and tension no matter the truth that there is no real hazard. This can bring about troubles which incorporates tension issues, put up-annoying stress sickness (PTSD), and phobias.

Scientists are despite the fact that analyzing approximately how the amygdala works, however they consider that it has a component in a whole lot of awesome techniques, along with:

Emotion regulation: The amygdala allows us to modify our emotions, which encompass fear, anger, and aggression.

Motivation: The amygdala urges us to avoid hazard and to are seeking out out rewards.

Memory: The amygdala allows us to encode and save memories of emotional occasions.

Overall, the amygdala is a complex and incredible thoughts shape that plays a key element in our emotional lives.

Here are some examples of ways the amygdala is worried in our normal lives:

When you spot a snake, your amygdala sends a signal to the relaxation of your mind, prompting the combat-or-flight reaction. This motives your coronary coronary heart rate to elevate, your breathing to turn out to be shallow, and your muscle companies to stiffen. This helps you to react swiftly to the hazard and to shield yourself.

When you're giving a presentation at artwork, your amygdala may also get active in case you feel apprehensive or agitated. This can purpose your voice to shake, your arms to sweat, and your mind to transport easy. However, if you can manipulate your anxiety, your amygdala can also allow you to perform nicely underneath strain.

When you observe a photograph of a cherished person who has passed away, your amygdala also can come to be active, causing you to revel in unhappiness and grief. This is a herbal reaction to loss, and it lets in us to process our feelings and drift on.

The amygdala is a powerful place of the brain, and it performs a essential characteristic in our emotional lives. By studying how the amygdala works, we're capable of discover ways to control our emotions more efficiently and to have happier and further healthy lives.

How does the amygdala reply to threats?

The amygdala responds to dangers in a completely fast and automated way. When the amygdala perceives a danger, it sends a signal to the relaxation of the thoughts and frame, prompting the combat-or-flight response. This reaction is characterized with the aid of the usage of numerous physical adjustments, which encompass:

Increased coronary heart fee

Increased blood strain

Increased respiratory price

Sweating

Muscle tension

Dilated scholars

The amygdala moreover performs a feature in emotional responses to dangers. When we experience a hazard, the amygdala releases strain hormones which encompass cortisol and adrenaline. These hormones put together us to combat or flee the chance, however they can also upward thrust to emotions of worry, worry, and fury.

The amygdala learns to partner precise stimuli with danger. For instance, when you have been bitten thru a canine inside the beyond, the amygdala can also discover ways to accomplice the sight of canine with risk. The next time you come across a dog, the amygdala may additionally elicit the combat-or-flight response, regardless of the truth that the dog isn't always clearly dangerous.

The amygdala is likewise worried in the creation of recollections of annoying events. When we undergo a trauma, the amygdala releases a surge of stress hormones. These hormones permit us to encode the memory of the trauma in order that we can avoid comparable occasions inside the future.

However, they can also make it hard to forget the trauma, even supposing we're strong.

Overall, the amygdala performs a key position in human survival. It allows us to quick and automatically reply to dangers. However, the amygdala additionally can be overactive, primary to tension issues, PTSD, and distinctive mental fitness ailments.

Here are some hints for coping with an overactive amygdala:

Identify your triggers. Once you understand what turns on your amygdala, you could begin to growth techniques for averting or managing them.

Practice rest techniques. Relaxation strategies in conjunction with deep respiratory, meditation, and contemporary muscle relaxation can assist to quiet the amygdala and reduce tension.

Challenge horrible mind. When you encounter an anxiety assault, it's miles essential to venture the horrible mind which may be going for walks thru your head. These views are generally unrealistic and unhelpful.

Seek professional help. If you are struggling to govern your anxiety to your non-public, please gain out to a highbrow health expert for assist.

How to reprogram your amygdala to answer a outstanding deal a lot less fearfully

To retrain your amygdala to respond much less nervously, you need to reveal yourself to the belongings you worry in a safe and managed environment. This method is known as publicity treatment. When you display your self for your anxieties, your amygdala learns that these items aren't definitely unsafe, and the fight-or-flight response is plenty an awful lot much less probably to be introduced on.

Exposure treatment:

Start via way of manufacturing a list of the belongings you worry, taken care of from least to most feared.

Start by way of method of disclosing your self to the least worried trouble in your listing. This have to require in reality considering the object, or it may contain often exposing yourself to it in actual lifestyles.

Once you are comfortable with the least feared item, pass straight away to the subsequent item to your listing.

Continue this approach until you have got uncovered your self to all the items for your list.

If you're afraid of public speakme, you will possibly begin through giving a presentation to a small organization of pals or own family individuals. Once you are cushty with that, you could attempt presenting a presentation to a larger accumulating of human beings.

If you're terrified of spiders, you can start thru looking at images

Mindfulness

Pay attention on your mind and feelings without judgment.

When you come across a daunting idea or feeling, renowned it without getting caught up in it.

Focus to your breath or at the contemporary moment that will help you ground yourself.

Cognitive restructuring

Identify the terrible ideals that result in your dread.

Challenge those notions by using way of the usage of asking your self if they may be sensible or beneficial.

Replace horrible wondering with extra sensible and useful thoughts.

Relaxation techniques

Deep breathing

Progressive muscular rest

Visualization

Meditation

These wearing sports can enable you to retrain your amygdala to reply much less nervously thru exposing you for your worries in a safe and managed environment. They additionally can help you to create more beneficial coping strategies for controlling your worry and tension.

Here are a few exclusive guidelines for reprogramming your amygdala:

Be affected character. It takes time and workout to change your mind's response to fear and tension.

Be regular. Do your sports activities activities continually to be aware blessings.

Find a guide gadget. Talk to a therapist, counselor, or sincere buddy or member of the family about your improvement.

Chapter 3: The Mind-Body Connection

The thoughts and frame are intricately intertwined. When we come across stress or anxiety, our our bodies respond with the useful useful resource of releasing chemical materials which consist of cortisol and adrenaline. These chemical substances put together us to combat or flee threat; however they can also make a contribution to a big range of physical symptoms, including extended coronary coronary coronary heart price, sweating, muscle tension, and complications.

Over time, continual pressure and tension can bring about a number fitness worries, in conjunction with:

Cardiovascular disorder

High blood pressure

Stroke

Diabetes

Obesity

Headaches

Digestive issues

Sleep troubles

Mental fitness difficulties which includes depression and anxiety

The particular records is that there are lots of things we are able to do to reduce strain and tension and enhance our popular fitness and well-being. Relaxation strategies together with deep respiration, meditation, and progressive muscle rest can assist in calming the body and mind. Exercise is likewise an great approach to alleviate pressure and lift temper.

Here are a few particular sports activities that you may exercise to relieve strain and tension and give a lift to the mind-frame connection:

Deep respiration

Deep respiration is one of the handiest and best techniques to alleviate stress and anxiety. When we breathe deeply, we set off the parasympathetic nerve device, that's responsible for our relaxation-and-digest reaction. This allows to sluggish down our pulse price, lessen our blood pressure, and loosen up our muscle tissues.

To do deep breathing:

1.   Find a snug role to sit down down or lie down with out troubles.

2.   Put your fingers to your stomach and your chest, respectively.

3.   Breathe gently and deeply through your nostril, feeling your tummy growth.

4.   Breathe out slowly thru your lips, feeling your tummy compress.

five.   Continue inhaling this manner for five-10 mins.

Meditation

Meditation is a topic that includes focusing your hobby at the winning second with out judgment. There are many terrific varieties of meditation, but they all entail taking note of your breath, your thoughts, or your frame sensations.

Meditation has been set up to provide diverse benefits for stress and tension, alongside side:

Reducing strain and anxiety

Improving mood

Improving sleep exceptional

Increasing pain tolerance

Reducing contamination

Improving cognitive characteristic

To meditate, sincerely pick out a quiet spot in which you could now not be troubled. Close your eyes at the equal time as you take a seat in a comfortable function. Focus your hobby in your breath. Notice the feelings of your breath getting into and exiting your body. Refocus your thoughts softly for your respiration each time they stray. Continue meditating for five-10 minutes.

Progressive muscular relaxation

Progressive muscle relaxation is a rest method that entails tensing and exciting every muscle organization in your frame. This method can help to relieve muscle tension and promote relaxation.

To acquire slow muscle rest:

1.   Find a cushty function to lie down in.

2.   Shut your eyes and take note of your breathing.

3.   Starting along aspect your ft, tension each muscle organization in your frame for 5-10 seconds.

four.   After tensing every muscle organisation, release it for 10-15 seconds.

five.   Continue tensing and exciting every muscle organisation for your frame, working your manner up from your ft in your head.

Exercise

Exercise is an top notch method to alleviate strain and enhance temper. Our our bodies launch endorphins during exercise, which could decorate our happiness. Exercise moreover facilitates to enhance sleep fine, which also can assist in decreasing pressure and anxiety.

On most days of the week, try to get in at least half-hour of mild-depth exercising. Any form of workout is wholesome, however a few endorsed opportunities encompass on foot, taking walks, cycling, swimming, and dancing.

By the use of those enjoyable techniques and exercising constantly, you may lessen stress and anxiety and beautify the thoughts-frame connection. This can motive a variety of fitness blessings, which includes multiplied mood, better sleep, and decrease danger of continual illnesses.

How pressure affects the body

Stress is a commonplace and often healthful emotion. It is the frame's natural reaction to risk or undertaking. However, even as pressure turns into excessive or extended, it can have a volatile have an impact on on the body.

Here is a primary examine of techniques pressure affects the body:

Cardiovascular gadget: Stress can produce an increase in coronary coronary heart charge, blood strain, and perspiration. This is because of the truth the frame is making ready to fight or flee the threat. Over time, persistent pressure can motive cardiovascular problems which includes excessive blood stress, coronary coronary heart illness, and stroke.

Digestive device: Stress can affect the digestive device, causing nausea, vomiting, diarrhea, or constipation. Acid reflux and heartburn also can end result from it.

Respiratory device: Stress can induce rapid respiration and shortness of breath.

Additionally, it'd make respiration situations like hypersensitive reactions worse.

Immune device: Stress can impair the immune device, making it greater difficult for the frame to combat off contamination.

Musculoskeletal gadget: Stress can cause muscle tightness and ache. Migraines and complications might also moreover give up end result from it.

Reproductive system: Stress can interfere with menstruation and idea. It can also growth the hazard of pregnancy issues.

Mental fitness: Stress can contribute to tension, sadness, and one-of-a-type highbrow fitness problems.

It is important to recognize that everybody reacts to strain in a notable manner. Some humans are greater inclined than others to the horrific consequences of strain.

If you're struggling excessive or non-forestall strain, it is crucial to make efforts to modify your strain tiers. There are severa alternatives to be had to you, together with:

Exercise regularly. Exercise is an first rate method to relieve stress and improve temper.

Get specific sufficient sleep. When you're nicely-rested, you're better able to address pressure.

Eat a nutritious food plan. Eating a first-rate food regimen can enhance your popular health and nicely-being, that would will can help you address stress more effectively.

Learn rest strategies. Relaxation strategies which includes deep respiration, meditation, and revolutionary muscle rest can assist in lowering pressure and boom rest.

Talk to someone you don't forget. Talking to a pal, family member, therapist, or counselor can permit you to approach your stress and create coping strategies.

If you're suffering to manipulate your strain in your non-public, please reap out to a intellectual fitness expert for help.

How to utilize rest techniques to relieve pressure

Relaxation strategies can be a very powerful approach to relieve pressure. They paintings with the resource of calming the frame and mind, and with the aid of manner of activating the parasympathetic nerve gadget, which is accountable for our relaxation-and-digest reaction.

Here are a few recommendations for adopting relaxation strategies to alleviate stress:

Find a peaceful region wherein you could no longer be .

Sit or lie down in a snug feature.

Shut your eyes and be privy to your respiratory.

Notice the emotions of your breath entering into and exiting your frame.

Refocus your thoughts softly in your breathing each time they stray.

Be affected person and everyday in your workout. It takes time and exercise to discover ways to loosen up deeply.

You can attempt the subsequent particular relaxation strategies:

Deep respiratory

Deep respiration is one of the most effective and simplest enjoyable techniques. To do deep respiratory, clearly take a look at the ones steps:

Put your hands in your stomach and your chest, respectively.

Breathe gently and deeply thru your nostril, feeling your tummy increase.

Breathe out slowly through your lips, feeling your tummy compress.

Continue breathing in this manner for five-10 minutes.

Meditation

There are many certainly one of a type varieties of meditation, however they all include focusing your interest on the prevailing 2d with out judgment. One easy shape of meditation is to focus for your breath. Simply study the ones tactics to carry out this:

Close your eyes on the equal time as you are taking a seat down in a cushty characteristic.

Focus your interest to your breath. Notice the feelings of your breath getting into and exiting your frame.

Refocus your thoughts softly in your respiratory whenever they stray.

Continue meditating for five-10 minutes.

Progressive muscular rest

Progressive muscle rest is a rest approach that consists of tensing and exciting each muscle organization in your body. This technique can assist to relieve muscle anxiety and promote rest. To accomplish contemporary muscle rest, take a look at those steps:

Close your eyes and lie down in a snug feature.

Starting along with your toes, anxiety each muscle group on your body for five-10 seconds.

After tensing every muscle institution, release it for 10-15 seconds.

Continue tensing and relaxing every muscle organisation to your body, strolling your manner up out of your ft in your head.

You can also try numerous relaxation strategies which encompass guided visualization, yoga, and tai chi. Experiment with terrific techniques to decide what works extraordinary for you.

It is vital to be patient and ordinary to your workout. It takes time and exercise to learn how to loosen up deeply. However, with everyday exercising, you may discover ways to exercise relaxation strategies to reduce stress and improve your elegant nicely-being.

Breathing physical games for rest

Here are some breathing strategies that you may try for rest:

Deep respiration

Deep respiration is one of the best and most effective interesting techniques. To do deep breathing, without a doubt follow those steps:

Close your eyes on the same time as you are taking a seat in a comfortable feature.

Put your fingers in your belly and your chest, respectively.

Breathe lightly and deeply thru your nose, feeling your tummy make bigger.

Breathe out slowly thru your lips, feeling your tummy compress.

Continue inhaling this way for five-10 minutes.

Alternate nose respiration

Alternate nose respiratory is a sort of pranayama or yogic respiration exercising. It is claimed to stability the left and right hemispheres of the thoughts and promote calm. To do change nostril breathing, check the ones steps:

Close your eyes whilst you take a seat in a snug position.

Place your proper thumb over your right nostril and your right index finger over your left nose.

Exhale out of your right nose and seal it collectively collectively together with your proper thumb.

Inhale out of your left nostril.

Close your left nose along side your right index finger and exhale via your right nostril.

Continue alternating nostrils for 5-10 minutes.

Lion's breath

Lion's breath is a effective breathing technique that is meant to remove pressure and anxiety. To do lion's breath, comply with those steps:

Close your eyes on the equal time as you're taking a seat down in a cushty characteristic.

Take a big breath and open your mouth full-size.

Stick out your tongue and curl it down.

Exhale forcefully thru your mouth, generating a "ha" sound.

Repeat steps 2-four more than one instances.

Bhramari pranayama

Bhramari pranayama, additionally known as bee breath, is a relaxing breathing exercise that is supposed to relieve tension and anxiety. To conduct pranayama, observe these steps:

Close your eyes even as you sit in a snug function.

Place your thumbs in your earlobes and your fingers over your eyes.

Inhale deeply through your nose.

Make a bee-like buzzing sound as you exhale.

Continue breathing and exhaling, generating a humming sound on each exhale, for five-10 minutes.

These are only a handful of the numerous absolutely one in every of a kind breathing strategies that you may hire for relaxation. Experiment with severa exercises to appearance what works satisfactory for you. You can also discover numerous guided breathing sporting activities on-line or in apps.

Progressive muscular relaxation

Progressive muscle relaxation (PMR) is a relaxation approach that involves tensing and enjoyable every muscle institution for your body. It is a clean and green method to lower tension and tension.

To do PMR, have a look at those steps:

Find a quiet vicinity in that you won't be careworn.

Close your eyes and locate a comfortable posture to lie down.

Take some deep breaths to lighten up.

Start with your toes. Tense your toes for five-10 seconds. Then, lighten up them for 10-15 seconds.

Chapter 4: Managing Difficult Emotions

Difficult emotions are a everyday a part of lifestyles. Everyone feels them from time to time. However, at the same time as hard feelings emerge as overwhelming or persistent, they may intrude with our each day lives and relationships.

Here are some thoughts for overcoming tough feelings:

Acknowledge your feelings. Don't try to repress or disregard your feelings. This will fine lead them to worse. Instead, word your feelings and take delivery of them for what they'll be.

Label your feelings. Once you've got got were given noted your emotions, try to categorize them. What emotion are you feeling? Is it anger, depression, worry, or something else? Labeling your emotions might also will let you understand them and assemble coping mechanisms.

Healthily precise your feelings. Once you have recognized your feelings, you need to discover a healthy manner to precise them. This might be speaking to a pal or member of the family, writing in a magazine, or indulging in physical hobby.

Challenge poor thoughts. Difficult feelings are regularly determined with the resource of unsightly thoughts. These mind is probably skewed and misguided. When you're feeling a painful emotion, confront your terrible mind. Ask your self if there is any proof to back your thoughts. Are you catastrophizing or leaping to conclusions?

Practice mindfulness. By concentrating interest on the triumphing second with out passing judgment, mindfulness is practiced. Mindfulness can allow you to grow to be more privy to your thoughts, emotions, and bodily sensations. When you're conscious, you can take a look at your emotions with out becoming stuck up in them.

Develop correct coping mechanisms. There are a whole lot of nicely coping techniques that could can help you manipulate tough emotions. Some examples include exercising, relaxation techniques, and spending time in nature.

Here are some more thoughts for overcoming particular difficult feelings:

Anger

Take some long breaths to relax.

Walk away from the situation if possible.

Talk to a person you accept as true with approximately the way you experience.

Engage in physical sports to discharge your rage.

Sadness

Allow your self to enjoy your disappointment.

Talk to someone you remember approximately the manner you experience.

Engage in sports activities which you revel in.

Spend time with cherished ones.

Fear

Identify the supply of your worry.

Challenge your terrible beliefs about the situation.

Develop a plan for managing your fear.

Seek professional assist if vital.

It is important to bear in mind that controlling tough feelings takes time and workout. Be affected character with yourself and do now not be scared to are attempting to find assist even as you need it.

What are tough emotions?

Difficult emotions are feelings which are tough to experience. They can be delivered on by using a multitude of occasions, which incorporates stress, loss, trauma, or infection. Difficult feelings can interfere with our each day lives and relationships, and that they can also cause physical and highbrow fitness problems.

Some examples of uncomfortable emotions include:

Anger

Anxiety

Depression

Fear

Frustration

Grief

Guilt

Shame

It is vital to understand that everybody reports painful emotions in each different manner. What one person thinks to be a painful emotion won't be difficult for a few different person. Additionally, the degree of painful feelings would possibly fluctuate from individual to person.

While hard emotions may be unpleasant and stressful to enjoy, they may be a normal a part of lifestyles. It is vital to recognize the way to govern difficult emotions healthily. By doing so, we are capable of lessen their detrimental impact on our lives.

Here are some thoughts for overcoming difficult feelings:

Acknowledge your feelings. Don't attempt to conceal or push aside them.

Label your feelings. What emotion are you feeling? Is it anger, depression, worry, or a few issue else?

Healthily particular your feelings. This can be speaking to a friend or family member, writing in a magazine, or indulging in bodily pastime.

Challenge horrible mind. Difficult feelings are regularly observed through the use of unsightly thoughts. These mind might be skewed and faulty. When you experience a painful emotion, confront your terrible thoughts. Ask yourself if there can be any evidence to decrease again your mind. Are you catastrophizing or leaping to conclusions?

Practice mindfulness. By concentrating interest at the winning 2d without passing judgment, mindfulness is practiced. Mindfulness can let you emerge as extra aware of your mind, feelings, and physical sensations. When you're aware, you can have a examine your feelings without turning into caught up in them.

Develop right coping mechanisms. There are quite a few top coping techniques that might will let you control difficult feelings. Some examples encompass workout, relaxation strategies, and spending time in nature.

Why is it essential to in fact accept your feelings?

Accepting your feelings is vital for various reasons:

It lets in you to understand your self better. When you acquire your emotions, you're accepting that they may be a part of you and that they're legitimate. This can permit you to better understand your motives, your triggers, and your modern day properly-being.

It permits you to method your emotions more correctly. When you try and repress or disregard your feelings, they tend to pile up and may sooner or later result in troubles together with stress, tension, and depression. Accepting your emotions permits you to gadget them healthily and bypass on.

It can enhance your connections. When you take shipping of your feelings, you are greater willing to be sincere with yourself and others. This can reason more potent and extra real relationships.

It can growth your intellectual fitness. Studies have verified that acknowledging your emotions may in all likelihood purpose greater intellectual health effects. For example, one take a look at indicated that oldsters who have been more accepting in their emotions have been a bargain much less possibly to broaden despair and anxiety.

Of path, accepting your emotions does no longer propose that you need to love them or which you want to provide in to them. It truly involves figuring out that they're there and permitting your self to sense them.

Here are a few guidelines for accepting your feelings:

Pay interest to your feelings. What feelings are you feeling? Where do you sense them in your frame?

Label your emotions. What is the word for the emotion you revel in?

Allow yourself to enjoy your feelings. Don't try and cowl or disregard them.

Be slight to yourself. It's good enough to enjoy uncomfortable feelings. Everyone feels them every now and then.

Practice self-care. Take care of yourself bodily and emotionally whilst you're going through tough feelings. This is probably consuming nutritious ingredients, getting nicely enough sleep, exercise, or spending time with cherished ones.

If you are difficult to truely get hold of your emotions, please attain out to a highbrow health professional for useful resource.

How to cope with tough emotions in a healthy manner

There are quite a few techniques to address tough emotions healthily. Here are some pointers:

Acknowledge and take delivery of your emotions. It's vital to allow yourself to experience your emotions, no matter the fact that they may be ugly. Trying to repress or forget about your feelings will simplest cause them to worse.

Identify the deliver of your emotions. Once what's producing your difficult feelings, you may start to enlarge coping techniques.

Challenge terrible questioning. Difficult feelings are normally located with the aid of terrible thoughts. These mind is probably skewed and faulty. When you're feeling low, confront your terrible thoughts through asking yourself if they're realistic and beneficial.

Healthily specific your feelings. There are numerous healthy strategies to specific your feelings, which encompass speakme to a chum or family member, writing in a journal, or undertaking bodily hobby.

Develop coping strategies. Several healthy coping mechanisms will will let you manipulate difficult emotions, which encompass exercise, rest strategies, and spending time in nature.

Here are some specific coping strategies that you may attempt:

Exercise: Exercise is an brilliant way to alleviate strain and decorate mood. On most days of the week, attempt to get in at least half of-hour of moderate-depth exercising.

Relaxation techniques: Relaxation techniques together with deep respiration, meditation, and revolutionary muscle rest can assist in quieting the frame and mind.

Spending time in nature: Spending time in nature has been showed to provide numerous advantages for highbrow fitness, which encompass decreasing stress, anxiety, and depression.

Talking to a person you accept as proper with: Talking to a pal, member of the family, therapist, or counselor can will can help you technique your feelings and create coping techniques.

Writing in a magazine: Writing in a magazine can be a extremely good technique to speak your mind and feelings and to track your emotional increase over time.

Engaging in sports you revel in: Doing subjects that you experience may additionally help improve your temper and decrease strain.

It is critical to broaden coping strategies that be surely proper for you and to try till you discover what allows you the maximum. There is not all of us-duration-fits-all approach for dealing with hard emotions.

Mindfulness bodily games for managing difficult feelings

Mindfulness sports can be useful for dealing with tough emotions because of the fact they teach you to be aware about your thoughts and emotions without judgment. This can assist you to turn out to be more aware of your emotions and to create coping mechanisms.

Here are a few mindfulness sports which you would likely try for coping with hard feelings:

Body test

A body take a look at is a mindfulness approach that consists of concentrating your interest on each location of your frame in flip. To take a body test, take a look at these steps:

1.   Find a cushty role to lie down in.

2.   Close your eyes and pay hobby your interest in your breath.

3.   Notice the sensations in your frame as you breathe internal and out.

four.   Starting at your ft, slowly direct your attention to every part of your body in flip.

5.   Notice any sensations you revel in in every phase of your body, which consist of warmth, coolness, anxiety, or rest.

6.   Don't criticize any of the sensations you experience. Simply notice them after which drift directly to the subsequent a part of your body.

7.   Continue analyzing your frame from head to toe.

8.   When you're finished, open your eyes and inhale deeply numerous times.

Mindful respiratory

Mindful breathing is a mindfulness interest that entails focusing your interest to your breath. To perform conscious respiration, observe these steps:

1.   Find a comfortable role to sit or lie down without troubles.

2.   Close your eyes and pay attention your hobby on your breath.

three. Notice the emotions of your breath stepping into and exiting your body.

four. Refocus your mind softly in your respiration on every occasion they stray.

Chapter 5: Changing Your Thoughts

Our mind has a wonderful impact on our feelings and behaviors. Negative mind can result in terrible emotions and behaviors, whereas happy mind can result in first-rate emotions and behaviors.

If you want to alternate your feelings and behaviors, you want to begin by using converting your wondering. This may be difficult, but it's miles feasible.

Here are some tips for changing your thoughts:

Identify your bad ideas. The first step to converting your thoughts is to understand your negative mind. What are the mind that run via your head on the identical time as you're feeling down, demanding, or irritated?

Once you've got placed your terrible mind, you may begin to combat them. Ask your self if your thoughts are practical and useful. Are you catastrophizing or jumping to conclusions?

Replace your awful questioning with more sensible and useful thoughts. As an possibility to wondering "I'm a failure," you could consider thinking "I made a mistake, but I can look at from it."

Challenge your horrible beliefs. Negative mind are typically based on negative ideals. For instance, if you consider that you are unlovable, you may have the concept "No one will ever love me."

To confront your terrible perspectives, ask yourself if there's any proof to guide them. Is there a few problem to your beyond that demonstrates which you are unlovable? Or, is it viable that your perception is based totally on a fallacious mind-set of truth?

If you find out that your horrible thoughts aren't supported through proof, you will likely begin to update them with extra powerful beliefs. For example, in choice to feeling that you are unlovable, you could bear in mind that you are well worth of love and admire.

Practice incredible self-talk. Positive self-communicate is the practice of talking to your self really and helpfully. It can permit you to increase your self-self perception and conceitedness.

To growth incredible self-speak, begin via noting the manner you speak to your self. Are you important and judgmental? Or, are you type and supportive?

If you discover that you are being vital and judgmental, query your bad thoughts and replace them with extra wonderful thoughts. For instance, in place of asserting "I'm so stupid," you could say "I made a mistake, however I can take a look at from it."

Focus on your strengths. Everyone has competencies and barriers. When you awareness for your strengths, you enjoy greater confident and cheerful.

Make a listing of your talents and abilities. Make a observe of this list and talk over with it frequently. When you feel low, take a glance at your list and remind yourself of all the belongings you are right at.

Practice thankfulness. Gratitude is the workout of spotting the great topics on your existence. It can will permit you to recognition at the wonderful and to sense more content material material.

Each day, take a couple of minutes to bear in mind the belongings you're thankful for. This may be some component from your fitness and own family to your career and hobbies.

Changing your mind calls for time and exercising. Be patient with yourself and do not become disheartened if you ride up on occasion. Just hold practising and ultimately, you'll start to understand a distinction for your thoughts, emotions, and behaviors.

If you're suffering to regulate your perspectives in your private, please reach out to a mental health professional for help.

How your mind have an impact in your emotions

Your feelings are significantly recommended by way of using your wondering. In fact, your mind can produce your feelings.

When you have got got a idea, your frame reacts to it with the useful resource of liberating numerous hormones and chemical substances. These hormones and chemical materials can lead you to feel cushty, unhappy, irritated, concerned, or each different emotion.

For example, when you have a questioning like "I'm going to fail this presentation," your body will release the pressure hormone cortisol. Cortisol should probable make you experience concerned and annoying.

On the opportunity aspect, when you have a questioning like "I'm going to do first rate on this presentation," your frame will release the texture-correct hormone dopamine. Dopamine may also make you enjoy assured and driven.

The greater you have got were given poor mind, the more your frame will release strain hormones. This can bring about chronic strain, that can have a unfavorable have an effect on on your physical and highbrow fitness.

The greater you have got got wonderful thoughts, the extra your body will release feel-exquisite hormones. This can cause a happier and greater healthy lifestyles.

Here are some strategies for harnessing your thoughts to create extra glad feelings:

Identify your horrible thoughts. The first step to improving your feelings is to pick out out the horrible ideals which might be developing them. Once what your horrible thoughts are, you can start to combat them.

Challenge your bad notions. Ask your self if your horrible beliefs are sensible and beneficial. Are you catastrophizing or leaping to conclusions? If so, replace your negative mind with more realistic and useful mind.

Focus on the terrific. Make a dependancy of focusing at the extraordinary additives of your life, whether or not massive or small. This will assist to teach your brain to consciousness on the coolest and to release greater revel in-relevant chemical materials.

Practice thankfulness. Gratitude is a powerful emotion that could help in raising your mood and improve your selected well-being. Develop the habitual of setting apart some time each day to reflect to your blessings.

Be affected character with yourself. Changing your thoughts calls for time and exercise. If you are making errors once in a while, do not give up. Just hold schooling and in the end, you will begin to apprehend a difference on your mind, emotions, and behaviors.

How to hit upon and challenge lousy thoughts

Here are some pointers at the way to find out and confront poor mind:

Identify your bad thoughts. The first step to addressing your horrific thoughts is to perceive them. Pay interest for your thoughts in some unspecified time inside the future of the day and word any thoughts which is probably awful, self-vital, or gloomy.

Journal about your perspectives. Keeping a mag is probably a superb method to recognizing your poor thoughts. Write down any ugly thoughts that you had all through the day, along aspect the scenario that provoked them and the manner you experience.

Challenge your terrible notions. Once you've got got were given decided your horrible thoughts, you can begin to fight them. Ask yourself the following questions:

Is this idea realistic?

Does this idea have any supporting evidence?

What is the worst that could arise if this notion had been actual?

What is the incredible that might take region?

What is the maximum in all likelihood state of affairs to arise?

Replace your awful thinking with greater realistic and amazing thoughts. For instance, you could agree with, "I'm organized for this take a look at and I'm going to do my great," in choice to, "I'm going to fail this take a look at."

Practice outstanding self-speak. Communicate with your self as you may a friend. Be courteous and supportive, and popularity to your skills and accomplishments.

It is vital to be affected individual and persistent whilst questioning your bad mind. It takes time and paintings to exchange your concept patterns. But with art work, you may learn how to count on more favorably and sense more awesome emotions.

Here are some different pointers for preventing poor thoughts:

Look for evidence to guide or disprove your thoughts. For instance, in case you are thinking "I'm no longer real sufficient," ask your self for evidence to assist this mindset. What are a few concrete examples of conditions if you have felt inadequate? On the other aspect, are you able to placed of any examples of times when you have succeeded?

Consider the ramifications of your thoughts. Are your terrible mind helping you or hurting you? Are they assisting you to acquire your goals or are they preserving you lower back?

Ask yourself in case your thoughts are low-priced. Are you catastrophizing or leaping to conclusions? Are you absolutely seeing in hues?

Challenge your assumptions. Are you making assumptions approximately your self or others that are not real?

Be compassionate towards oneself. Everybody once in a while has stupid thoughts. It's important to be kind to yourself and to definitely be given which you are doing the great you may.

Cognitive restructuring techniques

Cognitive restructuring techniques are a form of treatment that will let you pick out out and venture hard attitudes and beliefs. These techniques are based on the premise that your thoughts and beliefs have a profound effect to your emotions and behaviors.

By converting your mind and ideals, you may have an effect on the manner you feel and behave.

Here are some commonplace cognitive reorganization techniques:

Identifying poor ideas. The first step to cognitive restructuring is to perceive your negative mind. This can be finished through maintaining a belief mag or by way of in reality taking note of your ideas at some stage inside the day.

Challenging terrible mind. Once you have got got decided your terrible mind, you may start to fight them. Ask your self if your thoughts are practical and useful. Are you catastrophizing or jumping to conclusions?

Replacing horrible thoughts with extra fantastic mind. Once you have burdened your horrible mind, you could begin to replace them with more right mind. This may be completed thru seeking out evidence to guide your excessive notable views or with the useful resource of without a doubt focusing at the effective parts of the scenario.

Here is an instance of tactics to make use of cognitive restructuring techniques to confront a awful concept:

Negative perception: I'm going to flunk this activity interview.

Challenge: Is this concept sensible? Have I failed every venture interview I've ever had? Does this concept have any supporting proof? Or, is it practicable that I'm genuinely feeling worried about the interview?

Replacement idea: I'm organized for this project interview and I'm going to do my amazing. I actually have the competencies and enjoy that the business is looking for, and I'm confident in my skills.

Cognitive restructuring strategies may be beneficial for plenty of intellectual health issues, in conjunction with tension, depression, and placed up-annoying strain illness. They moreover may be effective for boosting conceitedness and handling difficult conditions.

If you're inquisitive about learning extra about cognitive restructuring strategies, please communicate for your therapist or counselor.

Mindfulness sports activities for converting your mind

Mindfulness wearing events can be effective for converting your mind via supporting you to end up extra privy to your mind and confront them in a non-judgmental way. Here are a few examples:

Thought labeling: This interest consists of simply tracking your mind and figuring out them without judgment. For example, when you have the idea "I'm going to fail this test," you could name it as "perception about failing the test." This can permit you to turn out to be greater aware about your thoughts and to understand them as separate from your truth.

Thought tough: Once you may label your mind, you may begin to mission them. Ask your self if your mind are sensible, beneficial, or accurate. For example, in case you get the wondering "I'm going to fail this take a look at," you could ask yourself if you have any evidence to lower back this concept. Or, you may ask yourself if this wondering is useful or inspiring.

Thought alternative: Once you have challenged your bad ideals, you could start to update them with extra fine and practical thoughts. For instance, you may take delivery of as genuine with, "I'm organized for this test and I'm going to do my best," in desire to, "I'm going to fail this check."

Here is an example of the manner to utilize mindfulness sports to modify a terrible perception:

Negative idea: I'm not right sufficient.

Thought labeling: Thought about not being unique enough.

Thought difficult: Is this idea sensible? What proof do I ought to assist it? Are there any examples of moments after I have been nicely enough?

Chapter 6: Challenging Your Behaviors

Our behaviors are generally inspired via our ideas and emotions. When we've got terrible thoughts or emotions, we are extra willing to participate in horrible behaviors.

For example, if you are feeling demanding, you may avoid social sports. Or, if you are feeling down, you could overeat or sleep too much.

The proper information is that we will alternate our behaviors with the useful resource of converting our mind and feelings. However, it is critical to recognize that changing our behaviors calls for effort and time.

Here are a few strategies for confronting your behaviors:

Identify your tough behaviors. The first step to enhancing your behaviors is to become aware of the behaviors that you need to alternate. Make a listing of all of the behaviors that you are not happy with.

Understand the placement of your trouble behaviors. Once you have were given recognized your hassle behaviors, you need to understand why you are sporting out them. What feature do they serve? For example, in case you keep away from social occasions because of the fact you are scared of being judged, your avoidance behavior gives a motive of maintaining you from feeling ashamed.

Develop change behaviors. Once you recognize the feature of your trouble behaviors, you could start to installation change behaviors that serve the equal function more healthily. For example, in choice to keeping off social interactions, you may often divulge yourself to social times and assignment your terrible perspectives approximately being assessed.

Set cheap desires. When you are trying to decorate your behaviors, it is important to create realistic desires. Don't attempt to regulate the whole lot straight away.

Concentrate on just one conduct at a time to start.

Make a plan. Once you have got set a cause, make a plan for a manner you'll attain it. This technique need to encompass steps which you need to take, in addition to resources that you need to hire.

Track your development. Tracking your development ought to possibly assist you to stay inspired and to recognize how an extended way you've got were given come. Keep a pocket ebook to record your progress and to discover any boundaries which you are having.

Reward your self. When you acquire a purpose, reward yourself. This will let you live brought on and to hold walking inside the route of your considered one of a kind desires.

Changing your behaviors requires time and artwork, however it's miles feasible. By following the ones suggestions, you could make the modifications which you want to stay a greater pleasing lifestyles.

Here are some other techniques for confronting your behaviors:

Identify your triggers. What are the matters that motive your tough behaviors? Once you comprehend what your triggers are, you may start to boom methods to govern them.

Develop amazing coping mechanisms. Several healthy coping techniques can assist you to regulate your emotions and keep away from conducting unwanted behaviors. Exercise, mindfulness practices, and amazing time with cherished ones are some examples.

Seek professional assist. If you are struggling to modify your behaviors to your private, please get professional help. A therapist can provide you capabilities and strategies for controlling your feelings and converting your moves.

Remember, changing your behaviors takes effort and time. Be affected man or woman with yourself and do now not emerge as disheartened if you adventure up once in a while. You'll in the end have a look at a difference in case you virtually hold walking in the direction of.

How do your behaviors have an effect in your anxiety?

Your behaviors ought to possibly have a primary impact for your anxiety. Certain conduct may additionally moreover worsen tension signs and symptoms and signs and symptoms, at the identical time as others can help to lessen them.

Here are some examples of behaviors which could worsen tension:

Avoidance: Avoidance is a traditional tendency amongst humans with anxiety. It includes warding off instances or devices that bring about tension emotions. While avoidance can deliver instantaneous respite, it could make tension worse in the long run. This is because avoidance maintains you from going via your issues and finding that they will be no longer as risky as you decided they may be.

Rumination: Rumination is any other regular tendency among people with anxiety. It includes focusing on terrible thoughts and fears. Rumination must make anxiety worse with the aid of retaining you targeted for your anxieties and making them appear greater actual and horrifying.

Perfectionism: Perfectionism is the belief which you ought to be perfect to collect achievement or well really worth of affection and apprehend. Perfectionism can contribute to tension because it imposes vain expectancies on yourself. It also can make you revel in worried about making errors, that can result in avoidance and rumination.

Substance use: Some humans use substances which consist of alcohol or tablets to deal with tension. However, substance use ought to probable make tension worse ultimately. This is due to the reality materials may want to have an impact in your mind chemistry and make you extra touchy to tension-frightening stimuli.

Here are some examples of behaviors that may help in relieving tension:

Exposure: Exposure treatment is a sort of remedy that includes frequently exposing yourself to the sports or items that purpose your anxiety. Exposure remedy can can help you understand that your concerns aren't as deadly as you agree with you studied they'll be and to create coping strategies for handling anxiety.

Relaxation techniques: Relaxation techniques along side deep breathing, meditation, and gradual muscle relaxation can assist in lessening tension signs. Relaxation practices can assist in quieting your body and mind and enhance emotions of properly-being.

Exercise: Exercise is an wonderful approach to relieve stress and anxiety. Exercise releases endorphins, which have temper-boosting outcomes. Exercise also can help in enhancing your sleep exquisite, which can also bring about a discount in tension signs and symptoms.

Social useful aid: Spending time with cherished ones and speaking approximately your anxiety can also permit you to sense better and to manipulate your anxiety signs extra successfully. Social assist can also permit you to accumulate new coping strategies and to experience plenty less by myself.

If you are preventing with anxiety, it's miles important to talk to a health practitioner or intellectual health expert. They will assist you to to apprehend the behaviors which can be contributing on your tension and set up a plan to regulate them.

How to apprehend and address avoidant behaviors

Avoidant moves are behaviors that you participate in to avoid a few factor that you dread or locate uncomfortable. While avoidant behavior can carry temporary respite, they can also make subjects worse in the long run. This is due to the fact avoidant movements save you you from going through your problems and know-how that they may be no longer as harmful as you located they may be.

Here are a few strategies for figuring out and confronting avoidant behaviors:

Identify your avoidant inclinations. The first step to challenge avoidant dispositions is to understand them. What are the matters which you avoid? What situations or people make you experience stressful? Once you apprehend what your avoidant behavior are, you may start to format a plan to cope with them.

Understand the feature of your avoidant actions. Why do you take detail in avoidant behaviors? What feature do they serve? For example, in case you avoid social conditions due to the reality you're scared of being judged, your avoidant conduct gives a reason of preventing you from feeling ashamed.

Challenge your lousy notions. Avoidant behaviors are usually based totally on horrible attitudes and beliefs. For example, if you keep away from social events due to the fact you're afraid of being judged, you could have the bad belief "Everyone is going to suppose I'm stupid." Challenge your poor ideals by way of way of the usage of asking yourself if they may be realistic and beneficial. Are you catastrophizing or jumping to conclusions? Is there any proof to manual your awful mind?

Develop change behaviors. Once you apprehend the characteristic of your avoidant behaviors, you can begin to set up possibility behaviors that satisfy the equal feature extra healthily. For instance, rather than heading off social interactions, you can step by step divulge your self to social instances and assignment your lousy views approximately being assessed.

Start small. It is important to start modestly whilst you are difficult avoidant behaviors. Avoid trying to acquire an excessive amount of too rapid. Start through making little goals for your self, which includes speaking to at the least one new character at a assembly or going to the grocery keep even as it is crowded.

Be affected individual. Challenging avoidant behaviors takes time and effort. Be patient with yourself and do now not turn out to be disheartened if you enjoy up every now and then. You'll ultimately be aware a distinction in case you just keep training.

Here are some special techniques for confronting avoidant behaviors:

Identify your triggers. What are the matters that reason your avoidant behaviors? Once you apprehend what your triggers are, you could start to extend techniques to manipulate them.

Create a assist device. Having a assist device of friends and family individuals who can encourage you to project your avoidant behavior can be very beneficial.

Reward yourself. When you venture your self and do some component that you are fearful of, praise your self. This will will will let you stay inspired and to hold strolling towards your goals.

Remember, addressing avoidant behaviors takes effort and time. Remember to be type to your self and persevere.

Exposure remedy approaches

Exposure treatment is a type of cognitive-behavioral remedy (CBT) that entails frequently exposing your self to the conditions or gadgets that purpose your tension. Exposure remedy is primarily based totally on the idea that by way of way of the use of dealing with your anxieties in a solid and controlled environment, you may learn how to manage your anxiety and lessen your avoidance behavior.

There are hundreds of numerous publicity therapy techniques that can be achieved. Some of the most typical strategies encompass:

In vivo publicity: In vivo exposure consists of little by little exposing your self to the horrifying state of affairs or item in actual life. For instance, when you have a worry of spiders, you could begin with the aid of the use of searching at photos of spiders, then looking films of spiders, and ultimately interacting with a actual spider in a consistent region.

Imaginal exposure: Imaginal exposure includes vividly envisioning yourself in a apprehensive condition or object. This may be performed the usage of guided imagery or simply with the aid of manner of shutting your eyes and envisioning yourself in the state of affairs.

Virtual truth publicity: Virtual reality exposure (VRE) employs virtual fact technology to create a simulated environment that exposes you to your anxious situation or object. VRE can be mainly beneficial for people who've phobias about matters which might be difficult or unstable to expose themselves to in actual existence, which includes heights or flying.

Exposure treatment may be used to treat numerous tension troubles, which includes phobias, panic disease, social tension disease, and generalized tension disorder. It additionally may be used to cope with placed up-demanding stress ailment (PTSD).

Exposure remedy is maximum a fulfillment while it is undertaken along a therapist. However, there are awesome self-assist publicity remedy packages handy. If you're considering trying exposure treatment in your very very own, it is vital to talk in your clinical health practitioner or intellectual fitness expert first.

Here are a few hints for schooling exposure remedy:

Start slowly. Don't try to show your self for your worst worry proper rapid. Start through exposing your self to a great deal less threatening situations and regularly paintings your manner as an awful lot as extra threatening situations.

Be regular. Exposure remedy works awesome even as it's miles practiced regularly. Aim to exercise publicity treatment for as a minimum half-hour a day, numerous times in line with week.

Stay comfortable. It is vital to keep comfortable on the identical time as you're mission exposure remedy. If you start to sense involved, take some deep breaths and try rest techniques collectively with innovative muscle rest or meditation.

Don't give up. Exposure therapy may be difficult, but it's miles crucial to stay with it. The more you display yourself in your problems, the masses lots less worrying you may experience approximately them.

Mindfulness bodily sports for wondering your behaviors

Mindfulness physical video video games may be powerful for tough your behaviors via way of allowing you to emerge as more aware of your mind and feelings and to create a extra accepting and non-judgmental thoughts-set within the course of them. This will let you in figuring out the triggers to your problem behaviors and putting in change, more wholesome techniques of coping.

Here are some physical video video games to exercise mindfulness:

Body test: A body check includes focusing your interest on each element of your body in turn. This can will let you turn out to be extra privy to physical feelings for your body, which can be beneficial for spotting triggers to your hassle behaviors.

Mindful respiratory: Mindful respiration entails focusing your interest to your breath. This can assist in calming the mind and body, and alleviate tension.

Thought labeling: Thought labeling is certainly recognizing your mind and figuring out them with out judgment. This can allow you to end up greater privy to your thoughts and to impeach unpleasant or unstable questioning.

Urge surfing: Urge browsing is a mindfulness approach that can be used to modify cravings and dreams. It involves monitoring your cravings and urges without judgment and letting them bypass with out giving in to them.

Chapter 7: Understanding Anxiety In Seniors

1.1 Definition and Types of Anxiety

Anxiety, a complicated and multifaceted emotion, manifests in numerous office work, affecting people specifically techniques. At its center, anxiety is an adaptive response, a sign from our psyche that heightens attention inside the face of perceived threats. However, on the same time as anxiety turns into chronic or disproportionate, it can disrupt the delicate balance of highbrow properly-being.

Definition: Anxiety, in its essence, is a country of uneasiness or apprehension, often accompanied with the aid of heightened physiological arousal. It encompasses some of emotional, cognitive, and bodily responses to expected threats, whether or now not actual or imagined.

Types of Anxiety:

1.   Generalized Anxiety Disorder (GAD): chronic and excessive worry approximately

everyday activities, regularly without a selected purpose. Individuals with GAD can also moreover discover it hard to manipulate their tension and might revel in physical signs and symptoms along with muscle tension and restlessness.

2.   Panic Disorder: Characterized with the aid of way of sudden, and intense episodes of worry, called panic attacks. These episodes can be located through physical signs and signs and signs like palpitations, shortness of breath, and a enjoy of drawing close doom.

3.   Social Anxiety Disorder: Involves an extreme fear of social conditions and a heightened feel of self-interest in social interactions. Individuals with social tension also can fear judgment or scrutiny, main to avoidance of social sports.

4.   Phobias: Specific and irrational fears of particular objects, situations, or activities. Phobias can result in avoidance behaviors and may considerably effect each day life.

five.   Post-Traumatic Stress Disorder (PTSD): Arises after exposure to a stressful occasion. Individuals with PTSD can also moreover additionally revel in intrusive reminiscences, nightmares, and heightened arousal due to the trauma.

6.   Obsessive-Compulsive Disorder (OCD): Characterized thru intrusive, undesirable mind (obsessions) and repetitive behaviors or intellectual acts (compulsions) accomplished to alleviate tension related to the obsessions.

Understanding the nuances of those tension kinds is important for developing tailor-made techniques and interventions to deal with the severa desires of human beings grappling with tension issues.

1.2 Prevalence of Anxiety in Seniors

The twilight years, often related to information and mirrored photograph, also may be determined through way of unique demanding situations, and anxiety is not any stranger to this diploma of life. The incidence of tension amongst seniors is an trouble of growing difficulty, as it can significantly impact their common nicely-being and fantastic of life.

Factors Contributing to Anxiety in Seniors:

1.   Health Concerns: Seniors might also grapple with continual fitness conditions, pain, or the uncertainty of age-related ailments, contributing to heightened tension stages.

2.   Life Transitions: Retirement, lack of a spouse or near friends, and the opportunity of expanded dependency can purpose tension as seniors navigate good sized existence adjustments.

three. Isolation and Loneliness: Social circles may additionally decrease with age, foremost to feelings of isolation and loneliness, which may be regularly associated with improved tension.

4.   Financial Stress: Concerns about fixed incomes, growing healthcare costs, and

economic stability in later years may be property of tension for seniors.

5.   Cognitive Decline: The fear of cognitive decline, dementia, or Alzheimer's disease can be a big deliver of anxiety some of the elderly.

Underreporting and Misdiagnosis:

An greater project in information the superiority of anxiety in seniors lies in underreporting and misdiagnosis. Seniors can also hesitate to speak approximately highbrow health problems due to stigma or the perception that emotional nicely-being is a herbal part of getting older. Furthermore, signs and symptoms of anxiety in older adults can occasionally be misattributed to physical fitness conditions, essential to under-analysis.

Importance of Recognition and Support:

Recognizing the prevalence of hysteria in seniors underscores the significance of enforcing strategies to promote highbrow health in this demographic. Increased recognition, recurring screenings, and fostering open conversations approximately highbrow well-being can make contributions to a extra supportive surroundings for seniors going through tension.

By addressing the specific demanding conditions and elements contributing to tension in seniors, we will paintings within the route of growing a extra compassionate and statistics approach to highbrow fitness in the later levels of lifestyles.

1.Three Common Triggers

Anxiety in seniors may be encouraged with the resource of way of a big variety of things, every appearing as a ability trigger that disrupts the touchy equilibrium of emotional well-being. Understanding those common triggers is instrumental in developing targeted interventions to alleviate tension and beautify the general highbrow fitness of seniors.

1. Health Concerns:

Chronic ailments, ache, and the uncertainty of managing fitness situations.

Fear of cognitive decline, dementia, or the improvement of modern fitness issues.

2. Life Transitions:

Retirement and the related shift in each day physical games and social dynamics.

Loss of a partner, close to pals, or circle of relatives individuals, primary to grief and loneliness.

three. Isolation and Loneliness:

Reduced social interactions due to physical boundaries, mobility troubles, or geographical separation.

Limited possibilities for engagement and connection in the network.

four. Financial Stress:

Concerns approximately constant earning, rising healthcare fees, and the financial implications of getting older.

Fear of becoming a burden on family people or going thru financial hardships.

five. Cognitive and Memory Concerns:

Anxiety arising from perceived memory lapses or the worry of growing cognitive issues.

Challenges in adapting to new generation or adjustments in cognitive abilties.

6. Loss of Independence:

Anxiety associated with a decrease in autonomy and self-sufficiency.

Reliance on others for each day sports activities activities and desire-making.

7. Social Pressures and Expectations:

Feeling judged or scrutinized in social situations, contributing to social anxiety.

Unrealistic expectations or societal pressures concerning growing older gracefully.

Chapter 8: The Impact Of Anxiety On Seniors

2.1 Physical Health Effects

Anxiety, regularly regarded as a condition specifically affecting intellectual properly-being, intricately weaves its effects into the cloth of one's bodily fitness, specifically among seniors. The complicated interaction between highbrow and bodily additives underscores the significance of spotting and know-how the bodily health consequences related to tension on this demographic.

1. Cardiovascular Impact:

Increased Heart Rate: Anxiety can reason the discharge of strain hormones, important to an improved coronary heart rate.

Hypertension: Prolonged tension may also furthermore make contributions to excessive blood strain, posing dangers to cardiovascular fitness.

2. Respiratory System:

Shortness of Breath: Anxiety may additionally reason speedy and shallow respiratory, leading to a sensation of breathlessness.

Respiratory Issues: Chronic anxiety may additionally additionally exacerbate gift breathing conditions, which encompass bronchial allergies or persistent obstructive pulmonary illness (COPD).

three. Musculoskeletal Effects:

Muscle Tension: Anxiety regularly manifests as muscle tension, contributing to stiffness and pain.

Pain and Aches: Persistent tension can exacerbate or make a contribution to musculoskeletal pain situations.

4. Gastrointestinal Distress:

Digestive Issues: Anxiety may also moreover purpose digestive troubles, collectively with nausea, stomach cramps, and changes in bowel conduct.

Appetite Changes: Seniors may additionally revel in modifications in urge for food, essential to weight fluctuations.

5. Sleep Disturbances:

Insomnia: Anxiety can disrupt sleep styles, essential to difficulties falling asleep or staying asleep.

Fatigue: Poor sleep high-quality can also result in daytime fatigue and faded physical energy.

6. Immune System Suppression:

Weakened Immune Response: Prolonged tension may also additionally suppress the immune gadget, making seniors greater susceptible to illnesses.

Delayed Healing: Reduced immune characteristic can avoid the frame's capacity to heal and get better.

7. Cognitive Impacts:

Concentration Issues: Anxiety may moreover bring about troubles in focusing and retaining hobby.

Memory Challenges: Chronic tension can make contributions to memory lapses and cognitive decline.

8. Impact on Chronic Conditions:

Exacerbation of Existing Conditions: Anxiety might also additionally worsen the symptoms of pre-gift persistent situations, complicating their manage.

Interference with Medication Adherence: Seniors experiencing tension can also moreover face annoying conditions in adhering to prescribed medication regimens.

Recognizing the bodily health effects of anxiety in seniors is crucial for holistic care. Integrating intellectual health problems into everyday healthcare techniques can result in superior first-rate of lifestyles, superior physical well-being, and a extra complete method to assisting the health of seniors.

2.2 Cognitive and Emotional Consequences

Anxiety, a complicated emotional u . S ., casts a profound shadow now not most effective over bodily fitness however furthermore over cognitive functioning and emotional properly-being, specially amongst seniors. Understanding the tricky interplay amongst tension, cognition, and emotions is important for imparting complete aid to human beings navigating the disturbing conditions of anxiety of their later years.

1. Cognitive Consequences:

Impaired Concentration and Focus: Anxiety can cause a wandering thoughts, making it hard for seniors to pay hobby on responsibilities and keep attention.

Memory Impairment: Chronic anxiety might also additionally contribute to reminiscence lapses and problems in recalling statistics, affecting each quick-term and lengthy-time period reminiscence.

Reduced Cognitive Flexibility: Anxiety can limit the potential to comply to new conditions, hindering cognitive flexibility and hassle-solving talents.

Negative Thought Patterns: Persistent anxiety also can foster poor belief styles, influencing perceptions and attitudes in the direction of oneself and the surrounding global.

2. Emotional Consequences:

Heightened Emotional Reactivity: Anxiety can make bigger emotional responses, leading to heightened reactivity to stressors and demanding situations.

Mood Swings: Seniors experiencing tension can be more liable to temper swings, with fluctuations among durations of tension and moments of emotional misery.

Increased Irritability: Anxiety can make contributions to heightened irritability, making it more difficult for seniors to navigate every day interactions with a sense of calm.

Feelings of Helplessness and Hopelessness: Chronic tension may additionally foster a feel of helplessness and hopelessness, impacting the general outlook on existence.

3. Interconnection Between Cognitive and Emotional Aspects:

Feedback Loop of Anxiety and Cognition: Anxiety and cognitive troubles can create a remarks loop wherein each exacerbates the opportunity, developing a cycle that can be tough to interrupt.

Impact on Decision-Making: Anxiety can cloud judgment and keep away from powerful choice-making, probable main to choices pushed with the beneficial resource of fear or avoidance.

Social and Interpersonal Effects: Emotional consequences of hysteria can have an effect on social interactions, contributing to social withdrawal, isolation, or strained relationships.

Understanding the cognitive and emotional consequences of anxiety in seniors is important to growing focused interventions that cope with both factors of well-being. By fostering a holistic technique to care, people, caregivers, and healthcare specialists can artwork collaboratively to useful resource seniors in reclaiming cognitive readability, emotional resilience, and a experience of peace in their every day lives.

2.Three Social and Interpersonal Impacts

Anxiety in seniors extends past individual opinions, weaving into the fabric of social interactions and interpersonal relationships. The complex dynamics between tension and social nicely-being among older adults show a complex interplay that warrants cautious hobby for holistic assist and intervention.

1. Social Withdrawal:

Anxiety may additionally lead seniors to withdraw from social sports activities and engagements, limiting their participation in network activities and interactions.

2. Isolation and Loneliness:

Persistent anxiety can contribute to feelings of isolation and loneliness, as seniors may additionally furthermore struggle to initiate or hold connections with others.

3. Strained Relationships:

Anxiety can take location in heightened sensitivity and irritability, probably straining relationships with family participants, pals, or caregivers.

4. Impact on Communication:

Seniors experiencing tension may also moreover additionally face challenges in powerful conversation, important to misunderstandings and difficulties expressing their mind and feelings.

five. Fear of Judgment:

Anxiety may additionally foster a fear of judgment or negative evaluation in social settings, inhibiting seniors from freely expressing themselves.

6. Reduced Social Support:

Social anxiety may additionally contribute to a reluctance to looking for assist from others, diminishing the critical feature of social networks in managing life's traumatic situations.

7. Interference with Daily Activities:

Anxiety can restrict seniors' capability to interact in normal sports, hindering their participation in pastimes, volunteer artwork, or awesome social pursuits.

8. Impact on Caregiver Relationships:

Anxiety should have an impact on the caregiver relationship, as seniors may additionally additionally furthermore grapple with emotions of dependency or worry approximately becoming a burden to the ones providing care.

9. Stigma and Misunderstanding:

Societal stigma surrounding intellectual health issues may also moreover exacerbate anxiety, main seniors to cowl their struggles because of fear of judgment or false impression.

10. Community Disengagement:

Anxiety may additionally moreover contribute to a reluctance to interact with the broader community, limiting seniors' revel in of belonging and connectedness.

Chapter 9: Identifying Anxiety In Seniors

Three.1 Recognizing Symptoms

Recognizing the signs and symptoms and symptoms of hysteria in seniors is a critical first step closer to offering well timed guide and intervention. As anxiety can show up otherwise in older adults, a nuanced statistics of these signs permits caregivers, healthcare experts, and seniors themselves to apprehend and deal with capability challenges to intellectual properly-being.

1. Cognitive Symptoms:

Excessive Worrying: Seniors may additionally experience persistent and uncontrollable worry about different factors of their lives, along side health, budget, or circle of relatives subjects.

Difficulty Concentrating: Anxiety can purpose problems in focusing and preserving hobby, ensuing in stressful situations with duties that require cognitive attempt.

Memory Changes: Changes in reminiscence, which includes forgetfulness and trouble recalling records, may be indicative of tension-associated cognitive outcomes.

2. Emotional Symptoms:

Irritability: Seniors with tension may additionally exhibit prolonged irritability, reacting more strongly to stressors and showing heightened emotional sensitivity.

Restlessness: Feelings of restlessness, an lack of ability to lighten up, or a feel of being on factor are not unusual emotional manifestations of tension.

Mood Swings: Fluctuations in mood, beginning from periods of anxiety and fear to moments of calm, can also furthermore signal emotional turbulence related to tension.

three. Physical Symptoms:

Muscle Tension: Anxiety regularly manifests as muscle anxiety, leading to stiffness, aches, and soreness, specifically within the neck, shoulders, and reduce once more.

Sleep Disturbances: Changes in sleep patterns, together with trouble falling asleep, staying asleep, or experiencing forced sleep, can be indicative of anxiety.

Gastrointestinal Issues: Digestive problems, which includes nausea, belly cramps, and modifications in urge for food, can be bodily manifestations of anxiety.

four. Behavioral Symptoms:

Avoidance Behaviors: Seniors can also furthermore showcase avoidance of sure situations or sports activities that motive tension, limiting their engagement in every day life.

Increased Dependency: Anxiety can bring about extended reliance on others for selection-making and every day activities, reflecting a fear of independence.

Social Withdrawal: Seniors experiencing anxiety can also withdraw from social interactions, proscribing their participation in network activities or circle of relatives gatherings.

5. Sensory Symptoms:

Hypersensitivity: Heightened sensitivity to stimuli, which encompass noise, mild, or touch, may be present in seniors with tension.

Difficulty Relaxing: An incapability to lighten up or revel in a revel in of calm, even in non violent environments, can also moreover endorse heightened sensory responses associated with anxiety.

Recognizing those symptoms requires a mixture of cautious commentary, open communique, and a willingness to cope with highbrow health issues. Early identity permits nicely timed aid and intervention, fostering a extra first rate trajectory for seniors grappling with tension.

three.2 Differentiating Anxiety from Other Conditions

Distinguishing anxiety from other situations in seniors is a nuanced technique that calls for careful interest of signs and symptoms and a entire records of numerous health elements. As positive signs and symptoms also can overlap with awesome medical or psychological conditions common in older adults, it's miles vital to differentiate tension from the ones capability options.

1. Depression:

Overlap in Symptoms: Anxiety and depression frequently percent symptoms and signs and signs and symptoms together with adjustments in sleep patterns, irritability, and social withdrawal.

Key Differences: While anxiety is characterized by means of way of way of immoderate worry and heightened arousal, melancholy usually includes continual emotions of disappointment, hopelessness, and a loss of hobby in or pleasure in sports.

2. Cognitive Decline:

Overlap in Symptoms: Cognitive decline, which incorporates reminiscence lapses, may be located in every tension and early levels of conditions like Alzheimer's infection.

Key Differences: Anxiety-associated cognitive signs and symptoms are frequently situational and might beautify with anxiety control, at the same time as cognitive decline has a tendency to be cutting-edge and irreversible.

three. Medical Conditions:

Overlap in Symptoms: Certain scientific situations, consisting of thyroid issues or cardiovascular problems, may also additionally show off signs and symptoms like advanced coronary coronary heart rate and fatigue that overlap with anxiety.

Key Differences: A thorough medical assessment is vital to rule out underlying bodily fitness troubles. Addressing those situations may additionally additionally alleviate associated anxiety symptoms.

four. Medication Side Effects:

Overlap in Symptoms: Some pills prescribed for physical fitness situations can also have facet effects that mimic tension signs and signs and symptoms.

Key Differences: Reviewing remedy lists with healthcare providers and thinking about adjustments or opportunity medicinal capsules can help choose out and manage treatment-brought about symptoms.

five. Chronic Pain:

Overlap in Symptoms: Chronic ache situations can also moreover furthermore contribute to anxiety-like signs, on the aspect of muscle anxiety and sleep disturbances.

Key Differences: Addressing and dealing with continual pain via pain manipulate strategies can also additionally alleviate associated tension signs and symptoms and symptoms and signs and signs.

6. Sleep Disorders:

Overlap in Symptoms: Sleep issues, together with insomnia or sleep apnea, can motive fatigue, irritability, and hassle concentrating—signs and symptoms and signs and symptoms additionally found in tension.

Key Differences: A sleep check or evaluation with the aid of a nap professional can help differentiate between tension-associated sleep disturbances and number one sleep issues.

7. Medication Withdrawal:

Overlap in Symptoms: Withdrawal from sure drug treatments, which includes benzodiazepines, also can result in tension-like symptoms.

Key Differences: A cautious assessment of drugs statistics and session with a healthcare issuer can help perceive and control withdrawal-associated signs and symptoms.

Differentiating anxiety from different situations in seniors requires a collaborative method regarding healthcare professionals, caregivers, and the human beings themselves. A whole evaluation, thinking about every bodily and intellectual health factors, permits for proper diagnosis and tailored intervention techniques.

three.Three Seeking Professional Diagnosis

While spotting signs and symptoms and signs and symptoms and symptoms and know-how ability differentials are crucial steps, the formal evaluation of anxiety in seniors is great executed via the expertise of healthcare experts. Seeking professional diagnosis guarantees an entire evaluation, correct identity of the unique tension illness, and the development of an effective treatment plan tailor-made to the individual's wishes.

1. Primary Care Physician Evaluation:

Comprehensive Health Assessment: A number one care physician will conduct a radical fitness evaluation, considering bodily fitness, remedy facts, and capability clinical conditions contributing to symptoms and signs and signs.

Diagnostic Interviews: Professional healthcare carriers often use diagnostic interviews to build up statistics about signs and signs and signs and symptoms, their period, and the effect on daily functioning.

2. Mental Health Professionals:

Psychiatrists and Psychologists: Mental fitness professionals specializing in the evaluation and treatment of intellectual issues can offer a more in-depth assessment of hysteria signs and symptoms and symptoms.

Psychological Testing: Psychologists can also additionally use standardized exams to diploma the severity of anxiety signs and symptoms and signs and pick out specific tension troubles.

three. Geriatric Specialists:

Geriatricians: Physicians that specialize in geriatrics can provide know-how in expertise the unique traumatic situations confronted through seniors, considering both bodily and intellectual health factors.

Geriatric Psychiatrists: Specialists in geriatric psychiatry are educated to deal with mental health troubles in older adults, along side the diagnosis and manage of anxiety issues.

four. Diagnostic Criteria:

DSM-five Criteria: The Diagnostic and Statistical Manual of Mental Disorders (DSM-five) offers requirements for diagnosing numerous tension troubles, assisting specialists make correct and standardized diagnoses.

Chapter 10: Lifestyle Modifications For Anxiety Reduction

Four.1 Importance of Physical Activity

In the pursuit of tension remedy for seniors, incorporating bodily pastime into their each day exercising workouts emerges as a powerful and multifaceted approach. The importance of carrying out regular exercising extends past bodily fitness, gambling a pivotal position in selling intellectual properly-being and primary great of life.

1. Stress Reduction:

Release of Endorphins: Physical interest triggers the discharge of endorphins, the body's herbal mood elevators, decreasing stress and promoting a experience of properly-being.

Cortisol Regulation: Regular exercising lets in alter cortisol stages, the hormone associated with pressure, stopping excessive production and mitigating the physiological effect of chronic pressure.

2. Mood Enhancement:

Improved Serotonin Levels: Physical hobby will boom serotonin production, a neurotransmitter related to temper regulation. Elevated serotonin degrees make contributions to a greater first rate and sturdy emotional usa.

Reduction of Anxiety Symptoms: Engaging in normal physical interest has been verified to lessen signs and symptoms and symptoms of anxiety, imparting seniors with a natural and to be had method of dealing with their emotional well-being.

3. Cognitive Benefits:

Enhanced Cognitive Function: Exercise has cognitive advantages, which incorporates advanced memory, hobby, and regular cognitive function. These upgrades can counteract the cognitive decline associated with ageing and anxiety.

Distraction from Negative Thoughts: Physical activity serves as a distraction from terrible mind and problems, permitting seniors to awareness on the present 2d and revel in a highbrow reprieve.

4. Sleep Improvement:

Regulation of Sleep Patterns: Regular workout contributes to the regulation of sleep styles, promoting higher sleep pleasant and addressing insomnia—an trouble often associated with anxiety.

Reduction of Restlessness: Physical activity facilitates burn up greater power, lowering restlessness and contributing to a experience of physical tiredness that aids in achieving restful sleep.

5. Social Engagement:

Community and Group Activities: Participating in employer bodily sports or community-based bodily sports activities gives opportunities for social interplay, reducing feelings of isolation and fostering a enjoy of connection.

Enhanced Social Well-Being: The camaraderie constructed via shared physical sports can decorate social bonds, growing a supportive environment that actually influences highbrow fitness.

6. Physical Health Benefits:

Cardiovascular Health: Exercise contributes to cardiovascular health, lowering the threat of coronary heart sickness and related conditions, which can contribute to anxiety in seniors.

Pain Management: Regular bodily interest can assist control chronic ache situations, addressing a common source of physical soreness and anxiety.

7. Empowerment and Independence:

Sense of Empowerment: Engaging in bodily pastime fosters a revel in of empowerment and control, permitting seniors to actively take part of their very very own nicely-being.

Maintenance of Independence: By selling physical strength and versatility, exercise facilitates seniors in keeping independence and autonomy in every day activities.

Incorporating physical interest into the lives of seniors is a holistic approach to anxiety comfort, addressing each the bodily and intellectual dimensions of properly-being. As a flexible and available device, exercise empowers seniors to take an active function in their intellectual health, promoting resilience and enhancing the general high-quality in their lives.

4.2 Nutrition and its Role in Anxiety Management

A well-balanced and nutrient-wealthy weight loss program plays a important position in selling highbrow health, and its effect on tension control is specifically outstanding for seniors. Proper vitamins now not high-quality helps physical properly-being however also affects neurotransmitter function, hormonal stability, and overall resilience to pressure, contributing to a entire approach to tension consolation.

1. Balanced Macronutrients:

Complex Carbohydrates: Foods like entire grains, end give up result, and greens offer a regular release of power and manual the manufacturing of serotonin, promoting a solid temper.

Protein Sources: Including lean proteins in the healthy eating plan, in conjunction with chook, fish, beans, and nuts, facilitates the synthesis of neurotransmitters and helps alter strength degrees.

Healthy Fats: Omega-three fatty acids determined in fatty fish, flaxseeds, and walnuts are related to stepped forward temper and cognitive feature, supplying vital vitamins for thoughts fitness.

2. Micronutrients and Antioxidants:

Vitamins and Minerals: Adequate intake of nutrients and minerals, which incorporates Bvitamins, magnesium, and zinc, allows the frame's stress reaction and helps modify temper.

Antioxidant-Rich Foods: Fruits and veggies wealthy in antioxidants, along with berries, leafy greens, and colorful greens, defend the thoughts from oxidative stress and infection.

three. Hydration:

Water Intake: Dehydration can exacerbate emotions of anxiety and fatigue. Seniors need to keep proper hydration levels to assist everyday fitness and nicely-being.

4. Blood Sugar Regulation:

Regular Meal Timing: Maintaining everyday meal instances permits modify blood sugar levels, preventing energy crashes which could make a contribution to feelings of irritability and tension.

Whole Foods: Choosing whole, unprocessed additives with a balanced combination of carbohydrates, proteins, and fat allows stabilize blood sugar stages.

five. Caffeine and Sugar Moderation:

Caffeine Intake: Excessive caffeine consumption can make a contribution to jitteriness and increased coronary heart fee, doubtlessly intensifying emotions of anxiety. Moderation is essential.

Sugar Control: Fluctuations in blood sugar ranges because of immoderate sugar intake can also contribute to mood swings and irritability. Choosing low-glycemic materials can assist hold solid electricity levels.

6. Gut-Brain Connection:

Probiotic-Rich Foods: A wholesome intestine microbiome is hooked up to intellectual fitness. Including probiotic-rich ingredients like yogurt, kefir, and fermented veggies allows gut health.

Fiber Intake: High-fiber foods make contributions to a wholesome digestive gadget, influencing the intestine-mind axis and likely impacting temper regulation.

7. Individualized Dietary Considerations:

Food Sensitivities: Some humans may be sensitive to certain substances, that might impact mood and standard properly-being. Identifying and addressing meals sensitivities may be useful.

Personalized Nutrition Plans: Working with a healthcare professional or a registered dietitian to make bigger customized nutrition plans primarily based on man or woman goals and choices.

8. Regular Monitoring and Adaptation:

Observing Dietary Impact: Seniors and their caregivers need to display how dietary adjustments have an effect on mood and anxiety signs and symptoms and symptoms and symptoms and signs and symptoms, adapting the nutrients plan as wanted.

Incorporating a nutritionally sound and well-rounded food regimen into the every day routine of seniors is an important detail of anxiety control. By nurturing the body with critical nutrients, seniors can help their highbrow health, beautify resilience to stressors, and make a contribution to an normal experience of well-being.

four.Three Adequate Sleep as a Stress-Reducer

Adequate and restful sleep is a cornerstone of intellectual and bodily nicely-being, gambling a pivotal role in stress reduction and tension control for seniors. Establishing healthful sleep patterns contributes to emotional resilience, cognitive function, and an standard experience of calm. Recognizing the importance of sleep is essential for seniors looking for treatment from anxiety.

1. Regulation of Stress Hormones:

Cortisol Regulation: Quality sleep allows modify cortisol ranges, the strain hormone.

Consistent sleep styles contribute to balanced cortisol secretion, stopping excessive stress responses.

Adrenal Restoration: During sleep, the adrenal glands recharge, ensuring they're organized to answer to stressors as it ought to be whilst big extensive conscious.

2. Emotional Regulation:

Mood Stabilization: Adequate sleep helps mood stabilization, assisting seniors method every day annoying conditions with a extra remarkable and resilient mind-set.

Emotional Processing: During sleep, the mind strategies emotions and consolidates reminiscences, contributing to emotional properly-being and a more balanced mind-set.

three. Cognitive Function:

Memory Consolidation: The consolidation of memories takes place in a few unspecified time inside the destiny of numerous levels of sleep, promoting cognitive feature and helping studying and memory.

Attention and Focus: Quality sleep complements hobby and consciousness, permitting seniors to navigate every day responsibilities with more performance and clarity.

4. Restoration of Physical Health:

Immune System Support: Adequate sleep helps a robust immune gadget, improving the body's capability to shield closer to ailments that might contribute to pressure.

Tissue Repair and Growth: Sleep is crucial for tissue repair, muscle growth, and regular bodily recuperation, contributing to most suitable health.

5. Sleep-Related Anxiety Reduction:

Nighttime Anxiety Management: Establishing a steady sleep routine and optimizing sleep hygiene can reduce middle of the night anxiety and sell a feel of calm earlier than bedtime.

Reduced Rumination: Quality sleep permits interrupt the cycle of disturbing thoughts and rumination, allowing the mind to reset and technique worrying situations with renewed mindset.

6. Sleep Hygiene Practices:

Consistent Sleep Schedule: Maintaining a everyday sleep time desk via using the usage of going to mattress and waking up at the identical time each day permits modify the frame's inner clock.

Optimal Sleep Environment: Creating a cushty and conducive sleep surroundings, together with a darkish, quiet, and funky room, supports uninterrupted rest.

Limiting Stimulants: Minimizing caffeine and nicotine intake, particularly inside the middle of the night, contributes to better sleep splendid.

7. Relaxation Techniques:

Pre-Sleep Relaxation: Engaging in rest strategies which incorporates deep breathing, meditation, or mild stretching in advance than bedtime can assist seniors unwind and prepare for sleep.

Mindfulness Practices: Incorporating mindfulness practices into the night habitual promotes a comfortable and focused mind-set, lowering anxiety and stress.

8. Seeking Professional Support:

Sleep Disorders Assessment: Seniors experiencing continual sleep disturbances must are seeking advice from healthcare specialists for an evaluation of ability sleep troubles.

Counseling and Therapy: Behavioral treatment and counseling may be useful for addressing sleep-associated tension and putting in location healthy sleep conduct.

Recognizing the profound effect of sleep on stress reduction underscores its significance inside the holistic technique to tension consolation for seniors. By prioritizing and optimizing sleep, older adults can beautify their emotional well-being, cognitive characteristic, and preferred resilience within the face of lifestyles's worrying conditions.

four.Four Mindfulness and Relaxation Techniques

Mindfulness and relaxation strategies offer seniors effective system to manipulate strain, lessen anxiety, and enhance ordinary properly-being. By cultivating present-moment recognition and promoting a experience of calm, the ones practices empower people to navigate lifestyles's demanding situations with greater ease and resilience.

1. Mindful Breathing:

Diaphragmatic Breathing: Seniors can exercise deep, diaphragmatic respiration through inhaling slowly through the nostril, permitting the stomach to boom, and exhaling lightly through the mouth. This promotes rest and reduces pressure.

Focused Breathing: Bringing interest to the breath and specializing in its rhythmic sample can function an anchor, supporting seniors stay gift and calm.

2. Meditation Practices:

Guided Meditation: Utilizing guided meditation recordings or apps can help seniors in reaching a rustic of rest. These intervals often hobby on breath consciousness, body scans, or visualizations.

Mindfulness Meditation: Seniors can workout mindfulness meditation with the beneficial aid of lightly bringing their hobby to the present 2nd, searching thoughts without judgment, and fostering a feel of recognition.

3. Progressive Muscle Relaxation (PMR):

Tension-Release Technique: Seniors can systematically demanding after which lighten up awesome muscle corporations, starting from the feet and progressing to the pinnacle. This method allows to launch physical tension and promotes a state of relaxation.

Body Scan: Conducting a body check includes taking note of every a part of the body, frequently fun muscle corporations, and letting drift of anxiety.

4. Yoga and Tai Chi:

Gentle Movement Practices: Engaging in moderate yoga or tai chi promotes bodily relaxation, flexibility, and mindfulness. These practices integrate motion, meditation, and breath.

Balance and Mind-Body Connection: Yoga and tai chi emphasize the connection a number of the frame and thoughts, fostering a experience of balance and calmness.

5. Visualization Techniques:

Guided Imagery: Seniors can engage in guided imagery bodily video video games, visualizing serene scenes or wonderful results to sell rest and decrease tension.

Nature Visualization: Imagining being in a peaceful herbal setting, at the aspect of a calming seashore or tranquil wooded place, can evoke a experience of tranquility and decrease stress.

6. Journaling and Reflection:

Gratitude Journaling: Encouraging seniors to preserve a gratitude journal can shift attention to splendid components of lifestyles, fostering a sense of appreciation and lowering stress.

Reflection on Positive Moments: Taking time to mirror on outstanding reviews and accomplishments can contribute to a more first-rate mind-set and emotional properly-being.

Chapter 11: Social Support And Connection

5.1 Building and Strengthening Social Networks

The energy of social connections is critical to the intellectual and emotional well-being of seniors, presenting a strong foundation for anxiety treatment and an advanced brilliant of existence. Building and strengthening social networks offers plenty of benefits that make a contribution to a experience of belonging, assist, and fulfillment.

1. Community Engagement:

Joining Social Groups: Seniors can explore nearby golf equipment, interest agencies, or network businesses to hook up with like-minded people who percent not unusual interests.

Volunteer Opportunities: Engaging in volunteer art work not most effective offers a experience of cause however moreover creates opportunities to construct big connections with others in the community.

2. Family and Friend Connections:

Regular Communication: Regular verbal exchange with own family and friends, whether or not or now not through telephone calls, video chats, or in-person visits, strengthens emotional bonds and fosters a manual tool.

Celebrating Milestones: Sharing within the birthday party of milestones, activities, and specific activities with loved ones creates a experience of connection and reinforces the importance of social relationships.

three. Technology and Social Media:

Virtual Connections: Embracing technology allows seniors to stay related with buddies and own family, mainly on the equal time as physical distance is a element. Video calls, social media, and messaging apps provide available way of communique.

Online Communities: Seniors can discover online groups that cater to their hobbies, fostering connections with individuals who percentage not unusual pastimes, opinions, or desires.

4. Seniors' Centers and Facilities:

Participation in Activities: Seniors' centers and facilities provide a number of sports, instructions, and events. Participating inside the ones programs offers opportunities to satisfy new humans and build friendships.

Support Groups: Joining useful resource organizations inner seniors' facilities can provide a platform to percentage studies, gather emotional assist, and assemble a sense of community.

5. Intergenerational Connections:

Mentorship Programs: Seniors may have interaction in mentorship applications with more younger humans, fostering intergenerational connections and supplying a feel of cause.

Family Gatherings: Encouraging interactions with more youthful family individuals, collectively with grandchildren, promotes a experience of continuity, joy, and shared testimonies.

6. Pet Companionship:

Pet Ownership: The companionship of pets has been confirmed to reduce strain and loneliness. Seniors can recollect adopting a puppy, presenting a source of unconditional love and companionship.

Pet-Related Activities: Participating in pup-associated sports, which includes canine taking walks corporations or puppy therapy training, can create opportunities for social interactions.

7. Continuing Education:

Enrolling in Classes: Seniors can discover academic possibilities, whether or not or no longer or not through formal training or workshops, to fulfill individuals with comparable interests and increase their social circles.

Book Clubs and Discussion Groups: Joining e-book clubs or speak agencies centered on subjects of hobby promotes intellectual engagement and social connection.

8. Open Communication:

Expressing Needs: Seniors should revel in snug expressing their social wants to pals, circle of relatives, or caregivers. Open conversation allows the improvement of supportive social networks.

Active Listening: Actively listening to others fosters deeper connections. Seniors can beautify their social interactions by using using surely engaging with others and displaying interest of their lives.

Building and strengthening social networks is a dynamic and ongoing technique that contributes drastically to the emotional resilience of seniors. By actively taking part in numerous social possibilities and nurturing large connections, older adults can create a robust help device that enhances their popular properly-being and lets in alleviate anxiety.

five.2 Family and Friends as Support Systems

Family and buddies play pivotal roles within the lives of seniors, serving as critical pillars of assist, know-how, and companionship. Nurturing the ones relationships now not great fosters a experience of belonging however moreover contributes considerably to tension treatment and not unusual emotional properly-being for older adults.

1. Emotional Support:

Open Communication: Creating an surroundings of open verbal exchange allows seniors to particular their feelings, concerns, and thoughts, fostering emotional connection and understanding.

Active Listening: Family and buddies can offer meaningful assist thru actively listening to seniors, validating their evaluations, and supplying empathy.

2. Shared Activities:

Quality Time: Spending remarkable time together via shared activities, outings, or leisurely moments strengthens bonds and creates great recollections.

Celebrating Achievements: Acknowledging and celebrating seniors' achievements, no matter how small, reinforces a enjoy of fulfillment and shared satisfaction.

three. Practical Assistance:

Assistance with Daily Tasks: Offering assist with each day responsibilities, at the side of grocery shopping for, own family chores, or transportation, demonstrates realistic assist and care.

Collaborative Problem-Solving: Involving family and buddies in collaborative trouble-fixing can alleviate stressors and create a experience of shared duty.

four. Regular Communication:

Scheduled Check-Ins: Establishing ordinary check-ins, whether or not or not thru cellular phone calls, video chats, or in-man or woman visits, keeps a regular connection and allows for the sharing of updates and concerns.

Sharing Life Updates: Keeping circle of relatives and friends knowledgeable approximately one's existence, studies, and pastimes ensures a sense of inclusion and involvement.

five. Celebrating Traditions:

Maintaining Traditions: Upholding circle of relatives traditions and developing new ones fosters a feel of continuity, shared records, and emotional connection.

Holiday and Special Occasion Celebrations: Celebrating holidays and particular activities together strengthens the bonds of family and creates a supportive and festive environment.

6. Inclusion in Decision-Making:

Involvement in Decision-Making: Including seniors in own family choices, even as appropriate, empowers them and reinforces their revel in of organisation and importance in the circle of relatives unit.

Respecting Autonomy: Respecting seniors' autonomy in desire-making, whilst presenting steering and manual, contributes to a revel in of control and independence.

7. Managing Transitions:

Navigating Life Transitions Together: Whether it's miles retirement, relocation, or adjustments in health, navigating existence transitions as a supportive unit allows alleviate tension and creates a feel of protection.

Family Meetings: Family meetings provide a discussion board for open discussions about vital topics, ensuring that everyone's views and issues are considered.

eight. Expressing Affection:

Verbal and Physical Affection: Expressing love and affection via phrases, hugs, and gestures enhances emotional connection and reinforces a experience of being cared for.

Creating a Supportive Environment: Cultivating an surroundings of affection and reputation inside the family and buddy circle promotes emotional well-being and tension bargain.

Fostering sturdy connections with circle of relatives and friends creates a reliable assist device that contributes extensively to the general happiness and intellectual health of seniors. By prioritizing these relationships and retaining a experience of connectedness, older adults can navigate the u.S.And downs of life with the assurance of a being concerned and supportive network.

five.Three Participating in Community Activities

Active involvement in network sports offers seniors not nice a feel of belonging but additionally valuable possibilities for social engagement, personal increase, and anxiety comfort. Engaging with the wider community fosters a colourful social life, contributes to ordinary properly-being, and affords a platform for constructing significant connections.

1. Community Groups and Clubs:

Joining Social Clubs: Seniors can discover and be part of community social golf equipment or hobby-based completely corporations that align with their interests, supplying a risk to meet like-minded people.

Book Clubs and Discussion Groups: Participating in e-book clubs or talk businesses encourages highbrow stimulation and lets in connections through shared pastimes.

2. Volunteer Work:

Community Service: Engaging in volunteer paintings in the community not first-rate contributes to the properly-being of others however moreover provides seniors with a sense of motive, accomplishment, and social connection.

Nonprofit Organizations: Volunteering with nonprofit corporations allows seniors to make a amazing effect, hook up with others who percent similar values, and expand their social circles.

3. Fitness and Wellness Programs:

Exercise Classes: Participating in enterprise workout education, which includes yoga, tai chi, or strolling companies, no longer best promotes physical health but moreover creates opportunities for social interaction.

Wellness Workshops: Attending wellness workshops on topics like nutrients, stress control, or mindfulness gives educational possibilities and a hazard to satisfy people with shared health desires.

four. Local Events and Festivals:

Community Festivals: Participating in community fairs, fairs, and sports offers a festive surroundings and possibilities to connect with friends and fellow community contributors.

Cultural Celebrations: Seniors can attend cultural celebrations or events showcasing network artwork, track, and traditions, fostering a revel in of network satisfaction.

5. Continuing Education Programs:

Lifelong Learning Courses: Enrolling in lifelong gaining knowledge of publications or workshops allows seniors to pursue intellectual pastimes, studies new abilities, and connect with pals who percent a passion for training.

Senior Learning Centers: Some corporations have reading facilities especially designed for seniors, presenting a supportive environment for persisted training.

6. Community Gardens:

Gardening Groups: Joining community gardening companies gives an possibility for out of doors hobby, reference to nature, and collaboration with fellow gardening fanatics.

Harvest Events: Participating in harvest events or farmers' markets creates occasions for seniors to showcase their gardening efforts and interact with the network.

7. Local Senior Centers:

Programs and Activities: Senior centers frequently host hundreds of applications and sports activities, consisting of enterprise nights, art work training, and social gatherings, presenting seniors with a dedicated region for interplay.

Chapter 12: Mastering Relaxation And Mindfulness

Enhancing Relaxation and Mindfulness Abilities

Relaxation techniques characteristic crucial system in preventing anxiety and worry By assignment those techniques, humans can prompt the frame's rest reaction, mitigating the bodily consequences of stress and anxiety. It is important to apprehend that relaxation is a observed potential that may be mastered over the years, allowing people to get entry to a country of calmness whenever crucial.

Deep Breathing:

Deep breathing proves to be a powerful rest method. By centering one's interest on gradual, deep breaths, humans can spark off the frame's natural rest reaction. Begin with the resource of finding a quiet region in which you can take a seat quite truely. Close your eyes and take a deep breath in via your nose, permitting your abdomen to boom truely.

Hold the breath for a few moments, then exhale slowly thru the mouth, feeling the anxiety leaving the body with each exhalation. Repeat this system numerous instances, steadily experiencing a experience of relaxation enveloping you.

Progressive Muscle Relaxation:

Another beneficial method is cutting-edge-day muscle rest (PMR). This exercise consists of systematically tensing and freeing precise muscle businesses to set off rest. Start via manner of finding a comfortable role, every sitting or lying down. Begin together together along with your feet, consciously tensing the muscle agencies for some seconds, and then freeing the tension, allowing them to completely lighten up Progressively art work your manner up via your frame, tensing and releasing each muscle organization, together with the legs, belly, chest, hands, and face. As you keep, consciousness on the feeling of rest spreading at some point of your body, relieving any tension or pressure.

Mindfulness:

Mindfulness serves as a few different effective approach for managing anxiety and worry. It consists of purposefully taking note of the triumphing 2d with out judgment. By cultivating mindfulness, humans can boom heightened recognition in their thoughts, feelings, and bodily sensations, permitting them to reply greater efficaciously to traumatic situations.

Body Scan Meditation:

One mindfulness exercising to don't forget is the body take a look at meditation. Find a quiet and snug region to sit down down or lie down. Close your eyes and convey your hobby to your breath, allowing your self to loosen up. Begin thru directing your attention on your ft, noticing any sensations or anxiety gift. Slowly pass your interest up thru your body, specializing in everybody issue and acknowledging any sensations or emotions without judgment. This exercising permits you to connect to your body, selling relaxation and a enjoy of grounding.

Daily Mindfulness Practice:

Incorporating mindfulness into your each day habitual can appreciably lessen tension and worry. Set apart a few minutes each day to engage in a mindfulness exercise, alongside facet conscious respiratory or a quick frame test meditation. By constantly working toward mindfulness, you can expand heightened self-popularity and beautify your potential to stay gift, even inside the direction of tough situations.

Learning to Embrace Uncertainty and Overcome Fear of the Unknown

Understanding the Fear of the Unknown:

Fear of the unknown arises from our desire for control and predictability. When confronted with unsure occasions, our minds will be inclined to assume worst-case situations and exaggerate capability dangers. This fear can display up in various factors of our lives, which consist of relationships, career choices, and everyday selections. However, it's far crucial to keep in mind that uncertainty is a natural part of lifestyles and that our fear of it's miles often disproportionate to the real dangers concerned.

Challenging Cognitive Distortions:

To discover ways to embrace uncertainty, it's far important to challenge the cognitive distortions that make contributions to our worry. Cognitive-behavioral remedy (CBT) offers powerful techniques to reframe our belief styles. By figuring out and questioning our awful mind, we can replace them with greater sensible and tremendous ones. This method facilitates us apprehend that uncertainty does not identical disaster and that we have the capability to govern some thing demanding situations come our way.

Assessing the Evidence:

One effective technique for handling worry of the unknown is evaluating the proof for and toward our annoying beliefs. Often, our tension is fueled via irrational thoughts and assumptions. By systematically analyzing the proof helping our fears, we will gain a more balanced mindset. This gadget encourages us to recollect opportunity effects and opportunities, in the long run lowering the intensity of our tension. Reflecting on beyond reviews can also provide reassurance that we've got got got effectively coped with uncertainty earlier than, reinforcing our capacity to deal with it inside the destiny.

Developing Coping Strategies:

Managing worry of the unknown entails developing powerful coping techniques. This includes carrying out behaviors that promote a revel in of control and safety at the identical time as accepting the inherent uncertainty of life. For instance, education mindfulness and meditation can assist us stay gift and reduce anxiety about the destiny. Setting realistic dreams and breaking them down into smaller steps can offer a based totally method to dealing with uncertainties. Seeking guide from relied on human beings or becoming a member of help organizations also can provide validation and know-how.

Gradual Exposure to Uncertainty:

Gradual exposure is a tested recovery technique for desensitizing ourselves to anxiety-scary situations. By intentionally exposing ourselves to barely unsure eventualities and step by step growing the level of uncertainty, we're capable of construct resilience and boom a greater tolerance for the unknown. This technique allows us to mission our anxiety and beautify the belief that we're able to successfully deal with uncertainty.

Chapter 13: Crafting A Strategy For Confronting Fears

Understanding the Concept:

Anxiety frequently arises from irrational fears, main human beings to keep away from those conditions. However, this perpetuates the cycle of anxiety, reinforcing the perception that the ones fears are insurmountable. The key to breaking this cycle lies in confronting fears via a scientific and gradual method.

Identifying Fear Hierarchy:

The initial step is growing a fear hierarchy. This entails figuring out tension-inducing situations and arranging them in order of growing distress. This permits people to systematically goal their fears, starting with pretty anxiety-horrifying situations and grade by grade shifting closer to greater tough ones.

Setting Realistic Goals:

It is essential to set sensible desires whilst facing fears. Striking a balance among pushing oneself and fending off overwhelming reviews is critical. By setting doable desires, human beings can experience a feel of achievement, boosting their self notion and motivation.

Implementing Exposure:

Exposure lies at the middle of this technique. It includes intentionally exposing oneself to anxiety-inducing conditions whilst preserving a revel in of manipulate and safety. This may be finished thru in vivo exposure, in which individuals confront feared conditions in actual life, or imaginal publicity, in which they vividly don't forget those conditions. Both techniques have tested powerful in reducing anxiety and desensitizing people to their fears.

Gradual Exposure:

Gradual publicity is important for the fulfillment of this approach. It includes starting with conditions that evoke mild to slight anxiety and frequently progressing to more difficult scenarios. This step-with the useful resource of-step method lets in people to construct resilience and benefit self perception as they conquer each diploma of tension. It is critical to move at a pace that feels hard however viable, making sure consistent and regular progress.

Utilizing Cognitive Strategies:

While managing fears, it's far critical to project and reframe unhelpful mind. Cognitive techniques help human beings recognize and modify distorted ideals that perpetuate anxiety. By changing terrible thoughts with extra practical and immoderate wonderful ones, humans can reshape their wondering styles and reduce tension ultimately.

Embracing Uncertainty:

Many anxiety issues revolve round the priority of uncertainty. By embracing uncertainty, humans can often relinquish the need for absolute manage. This consists of exposing oneself to situations in which uncertainty is present and practising reputation and tolerance toward ambiguous results. Over time, this fosters resilience and reduces anxiety related to the unknown.

Seeking Support:

Embarking on this journey on my own may be overwhelming. Seeking useful resource from loved ones or specialists can provide guidance, encouragement, and obligation. A help network also can provide reassurance in the course of difficult moments.

"The Impact and Universality of Anxiety"

Anxiety is a not unusual and frequently misunderstood emotion that could have an impact on everyone, no matter their social repute or achievements. In this bankruptcy, we find out the massive-ranging effect of tension and the manner it manifests in our lives.

At its center, tension is a natural response to perceived threats or dangers. It is our frame's way of protective us. However, in our modern-day international whole of regular stimulation, our brains have emerge as hyper-vigilant and susceptible to perceiving threats in which there can be none. This heightened united states of hysteria may be distressing and prevent our capability to feature correctly.

One charming aspect of hysteria is its ability to move past societal boundaries. It does now not discriminate based mostly on age, gender, or wealth. Whether you're a a hit authorities or suffering artist, anxiety can have an effect on anybody. It reminds us that we're all susceptible to its overwhelming unease.

Anxiety can take various paperwork, precise to every character. Some can also experience generalized tension disorder, characterized with the beneficial useful resource of chronic fear and worry, whilst others can also moreover face panic assaults or social anxiety. Regardless of its specific manifestation, anxiety can be debilitating and save you us from achieving our complete capability.

Additionally, anxiety now not best impacts our highbrow and emotional properly-being however furthermore our bodily health. Chronic tension can make a contribution to coronary heart disease, gastrointestinal troubles, and weakened immune systems. This connection some of the mind and body underscores the importance of addressing tension as a good sized problem.

In our fast-paced global, it is crucial to understand that tension isn't always a non-public failing or vulnerable factor. It is a herbal a part of being human, and we should try and apprehend and help people who revel in it. By fostering empathy and developing steady areas for open talk, we are able to lessen the stigma surrounding anxiety and paintings closer to locating peace of mind.

Although anxiety can revel in overwhelming, there may be choice. Many people have placed powerful coping mechanisms and remedies that permit them to manipulate their tension and stay alluring lives. From remedy and medicine to mindfulness practices and way of life modifications, there are various techniques available to navigate anxiety's complex maze.

In end, tension is a often occurring element of the human enjoy that impacts humans from all walks of lifestyles. By information its a ways-attaining impact and recognizing its universality, we are able to foster a greater compassionate and supportive society.

"The Complex Interplay: Genetics, Brain Chemistry, and Environment in Anxiety Disorders"

Chapter 14: Understanding And Combating Anxiety Disorders

Anxiety troubles are complex and numerous situations that deeply have an impact on the lives of tens of hundreds of lots of human beings. They are to be had in numerous paperwork, inclusive of generalized anxiety illness (GAD), panic ailment, and social anxiety contamination These issues can disrupt and debilitate humans, making it critical to understand and fight them correctly.

Generalized anxiety disorder, or GAD, is characterized thru persistent immoderate worry about normal lifestyles. People with GAD often discover themselves trapped in a cycle of catastrophic thinking, imagining infinite situations of potential disasters and dangers. This steady state of apprehension outcomes in bodily symptoms and signs and symptoms like restlessness, irritability, trouble concentrating, and disrupted sleep. GAD affects human beings irrespective of age, gender, or historic past.

Panic sickness, however, provides itself in every other manner. It consists of unexpected, excessive episodes of worry known as panic assaults. These attacks can arise with none smooth motive, leaving people feeling crushed and helpless. Panic assaults deliver terrifying physical signs and symptoms and symptoms like a racing coronary coronary coronary heart, shortness of breath, dizziness, and a enjoy of coming close to close to doom. In excessive instances, panic illness may also additionally bring about agoraphobia, wherein people avoid situations or places that would reason an assault, putting apart themselves similarly.

Social tension disease, moreover called social phobia, manifests as an excessive fear of judgment and scrutiny in social conditions. People with this sickness revel in overwhelming self-recognition that hinders their functionality to have interaction in ordinary sports activities activities. The worry of embarrassment or humiliation may be paralyzing, stopping them from speakme in public, attending social gatherings, or interacting with others. It is important to understand that social anxiety illness is going past shyness and considerably affects an person's ultra-modern properly-being.

It is clearly worth noting that humans can experience more than one forms of tension issues simultaneously, in addition complicating their journey within the direction of peace of mind. Compassion, staying electricity, and an data that everyone's enjoy is particular are vital even as drawing close those issues.

Fortunately, there are numerous treatment options available for human beings with tension issues. Psychotherapy, especially cognitive-behavioral remedy (CBT), has set up superb effectiveness in supporting human beings grow to be privy to and assignment horrific mind and behaviors related to tension. Healthcare specialists also can prescribe medicinal tablets like selective serotonin reuptake inhibitors (SSRIs) to relieve signs and symptoms.

In end, anxiety troubles are complex and severa. They embody numerous manifestations, from the persistent worry of generalized tension sickness to the sudden terror of panic sickness and the paralyzing fear of judgment in social anxiety disease. Recognizing the ideal techniques anxiety can appear is important in offering useful resource and effective remedy approaches. By acknowledging the complexity of those problems, we are able to foster empathy and equip individuals with the device and resources they need to navigate their private journeys inside the path of finding peace of mind.

Anxiety during History: Struggles of Influential Individuals

Throughout the a long time, anxiety has been a steady partner for masses splendid humans, highlighting the truth that this situation is extensively well-known. From well-known historical figures to influential personalities of our time, tension has solid its shadow over people from severa backgrounds and eras. This bankruptcy targets to shed light on the demanding conditions confronted via those people, imparting a glimpse into the huge-ranging impact of tension on human life.

Let us start with historic times, wherein even the fine conquerors of records were no longer proof against anxiety's grasp. Consider Alexander the Great, whose awesome army triumphs had been found by way of manner of way of a perpetual sense of unease and apprehension. Despite his notable achievements, Alexander lived in a country of regular fear, haunted with the aid of way of the possibility of dropping his empire or being betrayed by using his closest allies. His tension drove him to pursue navy conquests relentlessly, trying to shield himself from the vulnerabilities that plagued his thoughts.

Moving in advance in data, we come upon influential figures from the vicinity of literature who battled their personal anxieties. The famend Russian creator Fyodor Dostoevsky, appeared for his profound and psychologically complex novels, suffered from excessive anxiety for the duration of his life. Dostoevsky's anxieties often manifested as profound self-doubt and existential dread, challenge matters that permeate an awful lot of his artwork. His characters, too, grapple with the same overwhelming unease, presenting a poignant reflection of the writer's private struggles. Dostoevsky's potential to channel his anxiety into artwork is a testament to the profound effect this situation may have on innovative expression.

In more cutting-edge history, we find out influential leaders who, irrespective of projecting self warranty and electricity in public, confronted their personal battles with tension in personal. One such example is Abraham Lincoln, the respected 16th President of the united states. Behind his stoic outdoor lay someone forced through way of tension and bouts of despair. Lincoln's anxieties had been fueled through the large pressures of foremost a country torn apart thru civil battle. The weight of his alternatives weighed closely on his feel of proper and incorrect, and he frequently sought solace in writing letters to explicit his fears and doubts. Lincoln's conflict with anxiety reminds us that even individuals who appear invincible can be suffering from inner conflicts.

Beyond the realms of politics and literature, tension has affected influential individuals at some stage in numerous fields. The fantastic scientist Charles Darwin, for instance, skilled severe anxiety inside the direction of his life, specially in terms of his groundbreaking idea of evolution. The fear of public scrutiny and capability backlash from his buddies haunted him, fundamental to intervals of profound self-doubt. Despite those anxieties, Darwin persisted and left an extended-lasting impact at the scientific international. His evaluations feature a testomony that tension does no longer need to beat back one's achievements, but can alternatively gas non-public growth and resilience.

From Alexander the Great to Abraham Lincoln, and from Fyodor Dostoevsky to Charles Darwin, the struggles with anxiety confronted through the ones influential people spotlight the all-encompassing nature of this circumstance. Regardless of their region of information or the time wherein they lived, anxiety affected their lives, shaping their mind, actions, and legacies. By acknowledging the tension professional with the aid of such figures, we come to apprehend that this case isn't always limited to precise demographics, however as a substitute transcends time and societal boundaries.

This glimpse into the lives of historical figures grappling with anxiety serves as a powerful reminder that this situation can effect all of us, no matter their accomplishments or outward appearances. It requires us to domesticate empathy and understanding for people who war anxiety in our very very personal lives and acknowledges that, just like the ones humans, we too own the power to overcome our fears and reap greatness.

"Effective Methods for Managing Anxiety"

There are numerous powerful techniques for coping with tension, collectively with remedy, cognitive-behavioral remedy, and mindfulness strategies. Medications like SSRIs and benzodiazepines can help regulate neurotransmitters within the thoughts to reduce tension. However, it's miles critical to paintings with a healthcare professional for correct prescription and tracking.

Cognitive-behavioral remedy specializes in figuring out and hard awful idea styles that make a contribution to tension. With the assist of a therapist, human beings can learn how to reframe their mind and increase more healthy coping mechanisms. Exposure remedy, a part of CBT, consists of regularly confronting feared situations in a supportive environment.

Mindfulness strategies, rooted in mindfulness meditation, teach humans to be aware about the prevailing second with out judgment. By searching at thoughts and emotions without reacting to them, people can detach themselves from anxiety. Mindfulness-based definitely stress cut price packages may be beneficial in reducing anxiety and enhancing ordinary nicely-being.

It's critical to study that anxiety is a complex circumstance, and now not every remedy desire is suitable for every body. Some people may additionally additionally moreover require a aggregate of treatment alternatives or a tailor-made approach. Consulting with highbrow health experts is critical for assessing character needs and growing the right remedy plan.

In give up, there are numerous remedies and remedy plans to be had for dealing with anxiety, collectively with treatment, cognitive-behavioral remedy, and mindfulness techniques. By working with experts, people can discover effective techniques to regain manage over their tension and locate peace inside themselves.

Anxious Minds: Understanding, Challenging, and Overcoming

Understanding and Overcoming Anxiety: Types, Triggers, and Strategies

Understanding the numerous manifestations of hysteria and the triggers that supply upward thrust to the ones emotions is essential in developing effective strategies to control and triumph over them. By gaining perception into one-of-a-kind forms of anxiety, individuals can enhance their intellectual nicely-being and conquer stressful situations with self perception. This financial catastrophe explores the complex global of anxiety, highlighting its numerous office paintings and the underlying factors that make a contribution to their lifestyles.

Anxiety is not the equal for all and sundry. It is available in a unmarried-of-a-type paperwork, every with particular trends and triggers. Generalized anxiety sickness, for example, is characterised with the aid of chronic worry and excessive worry about different factors of life, often with none unique purpose. Understanding this form of tension permits humans to apprehend types of disturbing thoughts and adopt strategies to relieve their effect.

Another not unusual form of anxiety is social tension illness. People with this example revel in excessive worry and misery in social conditions, often because of the fear of being judged or embarrassed. By recognizing the triggers that incite those emotions, people can enforce coping mechanisms, which include deep breathing wearing activities or super self-talk, to navigate social interactions with more ease.

Specific phobias are each different class of tension. Whether it's miles a worry of heights, spiders, or flying, precise phobias elicit an remarkable worry response whilst faced with the object or situation. Understanding the perfect triggers lets in human beings to confront their fears regularly and the usage of techniques like publicity therapy or cognitive reframing to rewire their fear reaction.

Post-disturbing strain ailment (PTSD) is an anxiety sickness that could increase after experiencing or witnessing a disturbing occasion. Understanding the triggers that spark flashbacks, nightmares, or hypervigilance in humans with PTSD allows for the improvement of powerful coping strategies, collectively with grounding strategies or seeking out expert treatment, to address and manipulate those signs and symptoms and symptoms and signs.

Panic disorder is yet a few different manifestation of hysteria, characterised by using manner of the usage of unexpected and recurrent panic attacks. These assaults are frequently located through physical signs and symptoms and signs and signs inclusive of coronary coronary coronary heart palpitations, shortness of breath, and a feel of forthcoming doom. Identifying the triggers, which can variety from character to individual, empowers human beings to reply proactively and constructively on the equal time as confronted with an drawing near panic attack.

By gaining an in depth understanding of the wonderful types of anxiety and their triggers, individuals can increase powerful strategies to manipulate and triumph over their anxiety. It is essential to apprehend that everyone's experience with anxiety is particular, and what works for one person won't be as powerful for a few distinctive. This monetary break dreams to equip readers with strategies to enhance their mental well-being, irrespective of the correct shape their tension takes.

Furthermore, expertise the triggers that elicit tension allows people to proactively address the ones triggers in advance than they increase into overwhelming feelings. This may additionally contain imposing rest strategies, looking for help from cherished ones or experts, or carrying out activities that sell self-care and emotional well-being.

In give up, comprehending the superb sorts of anxiety and their triggers is vital in developing effective techniques to control and overcome tension. By gaining notion into the numerous varieties of tension and the elements that make contributions to their life, individuals can navigate via their tension with extra ease and self perception. Armed with this understanding, readers can embark on a journey towards improving their highbrow properly-being and attaining a sense of calm and liberation from tension.

Overcoming Cognitive Distortions to Reduce Anxiety

Recognizing and addressing cognitive distortions can be an effective tool in lowering anxiety and converting horrific concept patterns. By exploring the internal workings of our minds and statistics how our mind can misinform us, we are capable of regain control over our anxiety and create a greater enjoyable existence.

Cognitive distortions, also referred to as questioning mistakes or irrational beliefs, are the skewed techniques in which we interpret and recognize truth. They can turn out to be deeply ingrained, causing a consistent pass of bad mind and emotions. However, through turning into privy to those distortions and actively hard them, we are able to regularly weaken their hold on us.

One common distortion is "catastrophizing." This occurs even as we exaggerate the ability negative results of a scenario, blowing them out of percentage and seeing the worst-case state of affairs as inevitable. By spotting this distortion, we're able to query the validity of our catastrophic mind and counter them with greater realistic perspectives. This permits us regain manage of our thoughts in area of allowing them to spiral into anxiety-frightening styles.

Another commonplace distortion is "thoughts reading." This occurs at the same time as we count on we apprehend what others are wondering, often assuming terrible opinions or judgments approximately ourselves. By tough this distortion, we understand that our assumptions are not primarily based on real proof however as an opportunity on our very personal insecurities and self-doubt. This belief empowers us to are searching out explanation and have interaction in honest verbal exchange, lowering anxiety on account of misinterpreting others' thoughts.

Chapter 15: The Power Of Support

Developing a robust help gadget and attaining out for social support is crucial in overcoming anxiety. Anxiety ought to make us enjoy isolated and overwhelmed, however it's critical to bear in mind that we do no longer need to face it by myself. By actively trying to find and nurturing a guide network, we will find out consolation and strength throughout difficult instances.

Our help network can take many paperwork, such as information family contributors, compassionate pals, and professional therapists. They become our supply of guide, developing a safe vicinity wherein we are able to specific our fears and vulnerabilities with out judgment. They be aware about us and offer empathy, supplying comfort whilst we need it maximum.

Sharing our tension with others facilitates us lighten the burden we deliver and advantage new views. Our manual network can provide treasured insights, assisting us assignment our annoying mind and update them with extra rational ones. They offer exceptional viewpoints and suggestions that we might not have taken into consideration on our own.

Aside from emotional help, our assist community also can provide practical help. They can assist us navigate the method of looking for professional assist, accompany us to treatment periods, or studies effective remedy options. They remind us that looking for assistance is a signal of energy, not weak spot, and that we are now not on my own on this adventure.

Building a assist community takes time and effort, but the benefits are immeasurable. Start with the beneficial aid of attaining out to close family members and relied on friends, commencing about your tales. Creating an surroundings of openness encourages them to reciprocate and offer their help in move again.

Seeking social guide does no longer imply burdening others with our problems. It's approximately putting in place a mutual dating in which every events can lean on every unique within the route of tough instances. Just as we advantage from their empathy and understanding, we additionally have an possibility to resource them when they need it.

While buddies and circle of relatives provide valuable useful resource, it is also important to are looking for expert steerage while essential. Therapists, counselors, or anxiety guide corporations can equip us with coping techniques, deepen our knowledge of our state of affairs, and provide a revel in of belonging amongst folks who proportion similar memories.

Building a assist community takes time and staying strength. It calls for navigating the complexities of human relationships. However, the try we placed into fostering those connections will without a doubt pay off ultimately.

In conclusion, growing a aid community and searching out social guide is critical in overcoming anxiety. This community serves as a strong haven, presenting emotional assist, sensible assist, and alternative views. By nurturing those relationships and searching out professional guidance whilst desired, we will locate solace in facts that we're now not on my own on our journey to triumph over tension.

The Importance of Self-Compassion and Self-Care in Reducing Anxiety and Promoting Well-Being

Fostering self-compassion and working inside the route of self-care are crucial for decreasing anxiety and selling elegant properly-being. In a international that regularly expects perfection and places huge pressure on human beings, it's miles essential to prioritize self-compassion and self-care as essential pillars of our intellectual and emotional health.

Self-compassion includes treating ourselves with kindness, know-how, and assist, without a doubt as we would provide to a high-priced buddy going via a tough state of affairs. It approach acknowledging our non-public struggling and being mild with ourselves, in preference to harshly criticizing or judging our actions or feelings. By nurturing self-compassion, we're able to spoil free from the cycle of self-grievance and self-blame, which regularly make a contribution to anxiety and prevent non-public growth.

Practicing self-care is a key issue of growing self-compassion. It method tending to our bodily, emotional, and intellectual goals. Self-care is about spotting the significance of taking time for ourselves and engaging in activities that convey us satisfaction, relaxation, and rejuvenation. By prioritizing self-care, we are able to recharge our strength, lessen strain, and enhance our commonplace properly-being.

As we paintings toward self-compassion and self-care, it is vital to end up aware about and task any poor beliefs or self-communicate which could hinder our progress. Often, we maintain unrealistic expectancies for ourselves, questioning that we must benefit perfection in all areas of lifestyles. These unrealistic expectancies can result in tension and self-doubt. By questioning the ones ideals and replacing them with extra sensible and compassionate mind, we will cultivate a extra healthful mind-set that helps our well-being.

Furthermore, self-compassion involves embracing our imperfections and know-how that making mistakes or handling stressful situations is a natural a part of lifestyles. Instead of berating ourselves for perceived screw ups, self-compassion encourages us to view those reminiscences as possibilities for boom and reading. By adopting a growth attitude, we can method problems with resilience and self-recognition, in the long run lowering tension and improving our trendy properly-being.

www.ingramcontent.com/pod-product-compliance
Lightning Source LLC
Chambersburg PA
CBHW051725020426
42333CB00014B/1150